Echocardiography in ICU

Michel Slama
Editor

Echocardiography in ICU

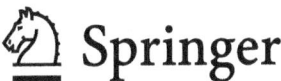 Springer

Editor
Michel Slama
Medical ICU
University Hospital
Amiens
France

ISBN 978-3-030-32218-2   ISBN 978-3-030-32219-9   (eBook)
https://doi.org/10.1007/978-3-030-32219-9

This Springer imprint is published by the registered company Springer
Nature Switzerland AG
The registered company address is: Gewerbestrasse 11, 6330 Cham, Switzerland

Preface

This book is designed as a useful pocket guide to echocardiography for the evaluation of hemodynamic failure. The authors consider critical care echocardiography to be the most important diagnostic and monitoring tool available to the frontline intensivist who deals with hemodynamic failure on a regular basis. Echocardiography allows the intensivist unparalleled capability to make immediate diagnoses, to direct initial and ongoing therapy, to measure key hemodynamic variables, and to serially monitor the hemodynamic function of the patient.

The text represents a cooperative effort between colleagues who have worked together on international guidelines on echocardiography, at conferences, at courses, and on research projects. Their combined expertise offers a practical and accessible guide for the frontline intensivist who uses echocardiography to guide diagnosis and management of the critically ill patient. The content emphasizes a pragmatic approach to critical care echocardiography with focused text that is accompanied by immediately applicable tables, figures, and algorithms. The electronic version of the book includes numerous cases and MCQ to challenge and educate the reader. We hope that this book will help our critical care colleagues to integrate critical care echocardiography into their daily practice to better manage their patients with hemodynamic failure.

Amiens, France   Michel Slama
New York, NY   Paul H. Mayo

Contents

Part I   TEE and TTE Views

2   Transthoracic Echocardiography: Views and Measurements 27
Stephen J. Huang

List of Videos[1]

[1]Electronic Supplementary Material is available in the online version of the related chapter on https://doi.org/10.1007/978-3-030-32219-9

Contributors

Daniel De Backer Department of Intensive Care, CHIREC Hospitals, Université Libre de Bruxelles, Brussels, Belgium

Stephen J. Huang Intensive Care Unit, Nepean Hospital, University of Sydney Nepean Clinical School, Sydney, NSW, Australia

Julien Maizel Medical ICU, Amiens University Hospital, Amiens, France

Paul H. Mayo Division Pulmonary, Critical Care, and Sleep Medicine, Northwell Health, New York, NY, USA

Anthony McLean Department of Intensive Care Medicine, Nepean Hospital, University of Sydney, Sydney, NSW, Australia

Sam Orde Nepean Hospital, Sydney, NSW, Australia

Michel Slama Medical ICU, CHU Sud, Amiens, France

Antoine Vieillard-Baron Surgical and Medical ICU, University Hospital Ambroise Paré, APHP, Boulogne-Billancourt, France

Philippe Vignon Medical-Surgical Intensive Care Unit, Dupuytren Teaching Hospital, Limoges, France

Inserm CIC-P 1435, Dupuytren Teaching Hospital, Limoges, France

Chapter 1
Ultrasound Physics

Stephen J. Huang

1.1 Characteristic of Sound Wave

Sound wave is a longitudinal wave where the particles vibrate in the direction of propagation. As sound waves propagate, alternate regions of *compression* (high pressure) and *rarefaction* (low pressure) are created. It is often easier to visualise sound wave as a sinusoidal wave with the peaks and troughs representing regions of compression and rarefaction, respectively (Fig. 1.1).

Sound waves are characterised by:

- **Wavelength** (λ), the length of one cycle
- **Frequency** (f), the number of cycles (vibrations) per second [unit: Hertz (Hz)]
- **Velocity** (c), the speed of the sound in a particular medium and depends on the 'stiffness' (B) and density (ρ) of the material
- **Amplitude** (A), which is proportional to the number of particles displaced and is related to loudness in sound; more power can move more particles, hence larger amplitude

S. J. Huang (✉)
Intensive Care Unit, Nepean Hospital, University of Sydney
Nepean Clinical School, Sydney, NSW, Australia
e-mail: Stephen.huang@sydney.edu.au

© Springer Nature Switzerland AG 2020
M. Slama (ed.), *Echocardiography in ICU*,
https://doi.org/10.1007/978-3-030-32219-9_1

1

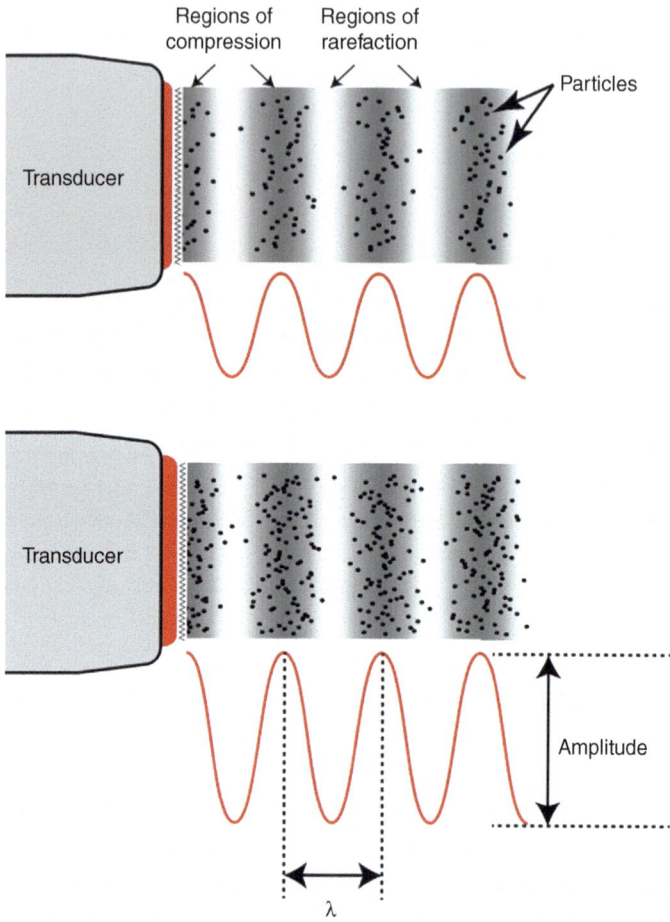

FIGURE 1.1 Sound wave

While λ and c change with the medium's density and 'stiffness', f remains constant regardless. Hence, wave is often being described by its frequency. Amplitude tends to decrease with the distance the wave travelled due to the dissipation of energy.

The relationship between f, λ and c is:

$$\text{Velocity}(c) = \text{Wavelenth}(\lambda) \times \text{Frequency}(f)$$

1.2   Diagnostic Ultrasound

The **frequency** of diagnostic ultrasound is typically in the range of MHz. For echocardiography, the frequency is 2–4 MHz.

In 2D imaging, ultrasound is transmitted in **pulses**, each consists of a defined number of cycles. The length of a pulse can be measured by the time needed to produce the pulse; this time is known as the **pulse duration** and is equivalent to transmission time. High frequency requires less time to produce one pulse; hence it has shorter pulse duration. After a pulse is transmitted, the transducer spends the rest of the time listening for echoes (**listening time**) until the next pulse is sent (Fig. 1.2).

The frequency by which the pulses are sent is known as **pulse repetition frequency** (PRF) and has nothing to do with ultrasound frequency.

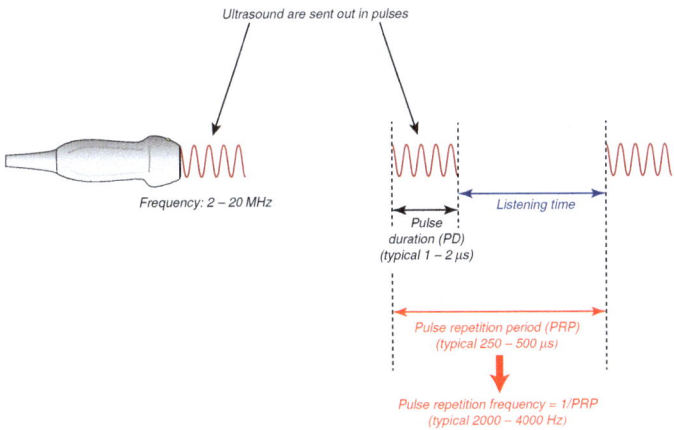

FIGURE I.2 Ultrasound pulse and pulse duration

1.3   Scattering, Reflection and Transmission

When an ultrasound pulse encounters a **reflector**, three things can happen:

- **Scattering**
- **Reflection**
- **Transmission**

1.3.1   Scattering

When the size of a reflector is smaller than λ (e.g. RBC), the ultrasound pulse is scattered in all directions. As a result, only a very small portion of echoes return to the transducer. Scattering gives rise to the characteristic acoustic appearance of the tissue (Fig. 1.3).

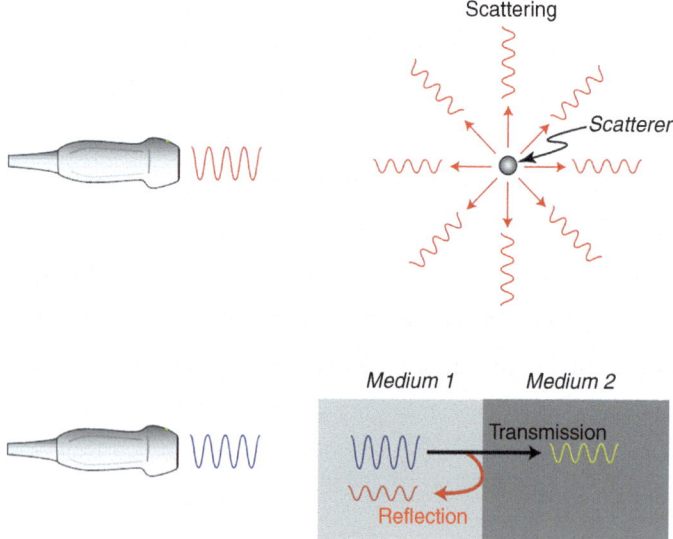

FIGURE 1.3 Scattering and reflection vs. transmission

1.3.2   Reflection

Reflection occurs at the interface of tissues where the densities are different. The larger is the difference, the more ultrasound is reflected. Near total reflection occurs at air-tissue interface explaining why lung, with multiple air-tissue interfaces, is a poor ultrasound conductor (Fig. 1.3).

1.3.3   Transmission

Ultrasound that is not reflected will continue to travel across the tissue boundary (transmission) (Fig. 1.3). Tissues of similar densities favour transmission than reflection.

1.4   Attenuation

Ultrasound energy, hence amplitude, gradually diminishes as the ultrasound pulse penetrates deeper into the tissue. This phenomenon is known as **attenuation**. The loss of energy can be due to three main reasons (Fig. 1.4):

1. **Scattering** where energy is reflected in all directions (see above)
2. Overcoming **tissue viscosity** (stiffness or resistance) where energy is lost as heat
3. **Reflections** hence less energy available for penetration

As a result, the amplitude of the transmitted pulse is reduced, and the image brightness is also reduced with depth.

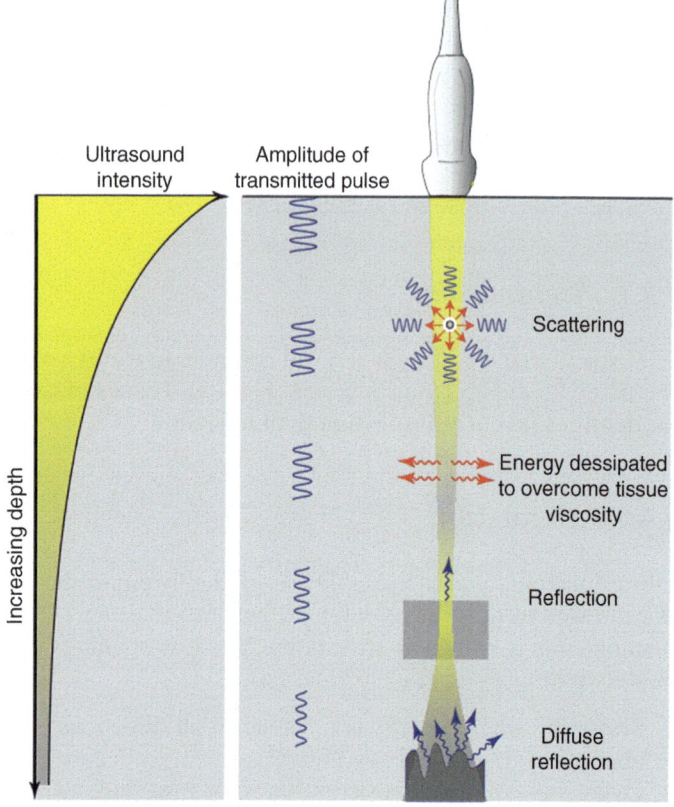

FIGURE 1.4 Attenuation

✱✱Practical Tips

How to improve brightness at deeper structures

1. Increase the far-field gain using **time gain compensation** (TGC).
2. Position the **focal point** at the far field.
3. Lower the **frequency** to minimise energy loss and to increase penetration.
4. Activate **tissue harmonic imaging** (THI).

1.5   Beam Focusing and Lateral Resolution

1.5.1   Beam Focusing

Electronic focusing is normally deployed in modern trans-
ducers. During focusing, the ultrasound beam converges
toward a **focal zone**. The focal zone has the narrowest beam
width and the highest beam intensity (Fig. 1.5).

1.5.2   Lateral Resolution

The ability to resolve two reflectors lying side by side is
known as **lateral resolution**. To resolve two closely placed
reflectors, the beam width needs to be narrower than the

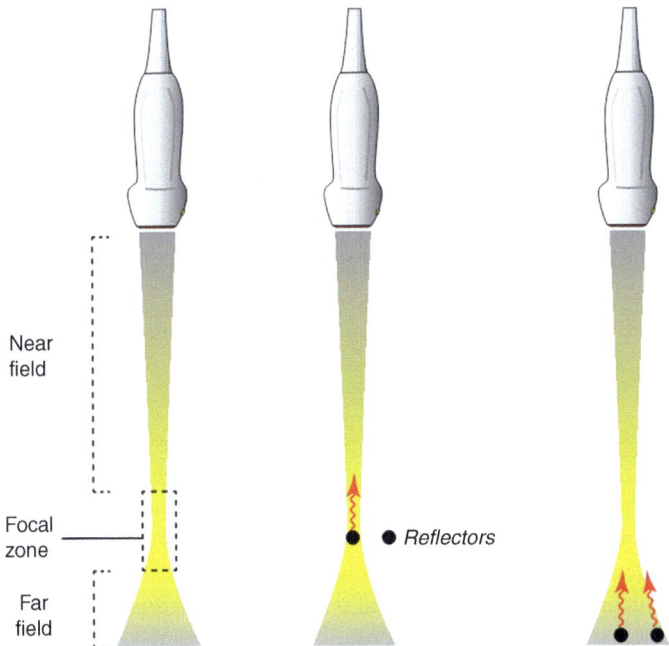

Near
field

Focal
zone

Far
field

● Reflectors

FIGURE 1.5 Beam focusing and lateral resolution

distance between the two reflectors such that each reflector sends an echo back to the transducer at different times.

If two reflectors send echoes back to the transducer at the same time, the ultrasound machine will not be able to tell (resolve) that there are two different reflectors. This happens when the two reflectors are not lying in the focal zone. As a result, the lateral resolution is compromised (Fig. 1.5).

**Practical Tips

- Focus position adjustment is available in most machines. Adjust the focus position to the level where you want the best resolution, e.g. vegetation.
- Some machine provides dual focus, but this will compromise the frame rate.

1.6   Frequency, Pulse Duration and Axial Resolution

1.6.1   Frequency and Pulse Duration

With the same number of cycles in each pulse, **high frequency** results in shorter **pulse duration** (PD), i.e. shorter pulse (Fig. 1.2).

1.6.2   Axial Resolution

The ability to resolve two reflectors arranged vertically (in the direction of the beam) is known as **axial resolution**.

Axial resolution depends on the pulse duration (or pulse length) (Fig. 1.6). When a pulse reaches an interface (first reflector), part of the ultrasound will be reflected (first echo, blue arrow in the figure) and the rest will be transmitted (yellow arrow). If the transmitted pulse encounters a second interface, some of the ultrasound will again be reflected (second echo).

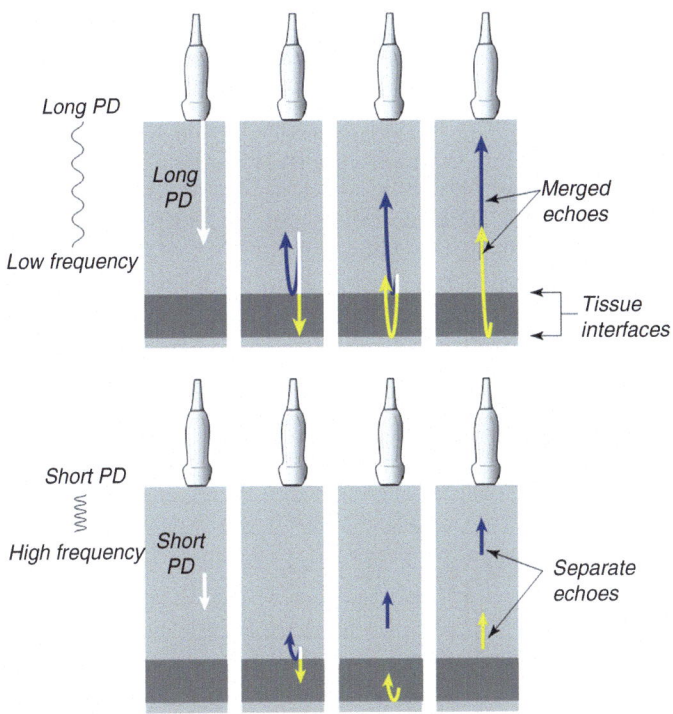

FIGURE 1.6 Pulse duration and axial resolution

If the PD is long, the second echo may catch up with the first echo and be merged with it, resulting in one single long echo, i.e. one broad interface instead of two separate interfaces.

If the PD is short, the first echo will be completely separated from the second echo, resulting in two separate signals.

＊＊**Practical Tips**

Use high frequency for better image. However, if the patient is big (obese), low frequency may produce better image due to better **penetration**.

1.7   Dynamic Range

A 2D ultrasound image is represented by shades of gray. Different structures have different shades of gray (Fig. 1.7). These shades of gray can be modified by changing the range of the original scale to another one, either wider or narrower. **Dynamic range** (DR) describes how the original range of gray scale is displayed. For example, if the range is 'compressed' (reduced DR), the structure with lighter gray and darker gray will appear as white and dark, respectively. This results in an image with higher contrast, i.e. more black and white. On the other hand, a wider DR image appears 'softer'. Some machines use the term '**compression**' instead of 'dynamic range' (Fig. 1.7).

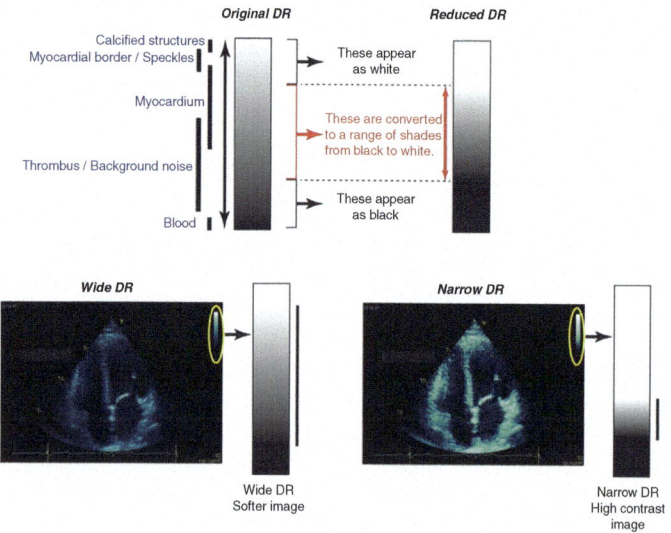

FIGURE 1.7 Dynamic range and its effect on image quality

Practical Tips

Narrow DR
- To eliminate low-level background noise but enhances the cardiac structures, that is, increases the contrast.
- Good for border detection; hence it helps in measurements.

Wide DR
- Brings out the weaker signals.
- Results in softer images.
- Best for detecting structures with little echo variation, such as thrombus, vegetation and tumor.

1.8   Doppler Echocardiography

1.8.1   Doppler Echocardiography

Doppler echocardiography can be used to measure blood flow velocity, as well as tissue velocity. As a reflector (e.g. RBCs) moves towards or away from the transducer, it changes the reflected ultrasound (echo) frequency. The echo frequency (f_r) is higher than the original transmitted frequency (f_o) when the reflector is moving towards the transducer and is lower when moving away. The machine calculates the velocity from the **Doppler shift**, defined as the difference between the transmitted frequency and echo frequency $(f_o - f_r)$ (Fig. 1.8).

1.8.2   Pulsed-Wave (PW) Doppler

As in 2D echo, PW Doppler utilises ultrasound pulses. Using the **sample volume** (gate), the operator can choose the location of measurement.

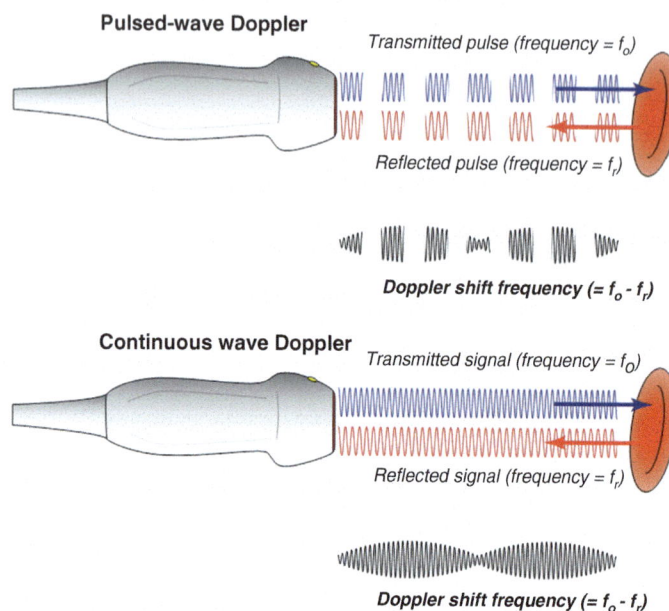

FIGURE 1.8 Pulsed-wave and continuous-wave Doppler

1.8.3   Continuous Wave (CW) Doppler

The transducer transmits and receives ultrasound continuously. All echoes along the beam path will be received and interrogated. Hence, the operator cannot choose the location of measurement.

∗∗Practical Tips

- Use PW Doppler to measure **low-velocity (e.g. ≤1.7 m/s) signal** and when you want to measure the velocity at a specific location.
- Use CW Doppler to measure **high-velocity (e.g. ≥1.7 m/s) flow**, e.g. regurgitant or stenotic flows.

1.9   Useful Doppler Measurements

1.9.1   Peak Velocity

The peak velocity (v) is used to calculate the transvalvular pressure gradient (ΔP) using the **simplified Bernoulli equation** (SBE):

$$\Delta P = 4\left(v - v_0\right)^2 = 4v^2$$

SBE assumes that proximal velocity (v_0) is zero, and v is the velocity at vena contracta. Peak velocity is used in estimating pulmonary artery pressures or ΔP in dynamic outflow obstruction (Fig. 1.9).

1.9.2   Velocity Time Integral

Velocity time integral (VTI), the area under the velocity curve (Doppler spectrum), is obtained by tracing the spectrum for a single beat (Fig. 1.9). VTI represents the total velocity obtained for a single beat and is useful in two aspects.

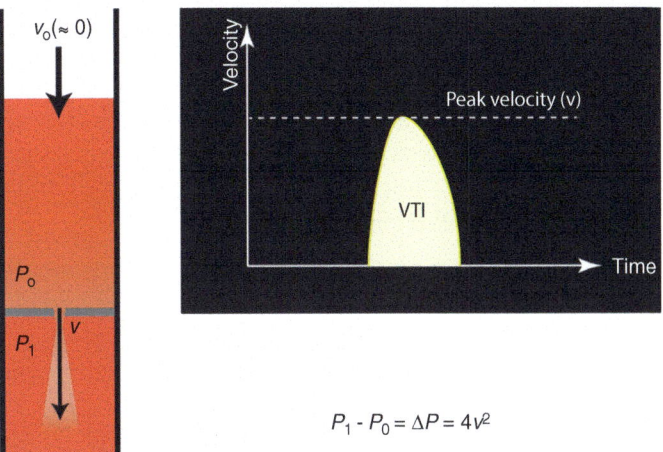

$$P_1 - P_0 = \Delta P = 4v^2$$

FIGURE 1.9 Peak velocity and velocity time integral

1.9.2.1   Calculation of Volumetric Flow

Volumetric flow, such as stroke volume, can be obtained by multiplying the VTI with the cross-sectional area (CSA). Hence, if the left ventricular outflow tract's (LVOT) diameter (d) and velocity (V_{LVOT}) is measured, then the stroke volume is

$$\text{Stroke volume} = \text{CSA} \times V_{LVOT} = \pi \left(\frac{d}{2} \right)^2 \times V_{LVOT}$$

1.9.2.2   Calculation of Mean Pressure Gradient

Mean ΔP is sometimes used to quantify the severity of valvular disease, such as aortic stenosis. It is obtained by tracing the Doppler spectrum, and the machine will automatically calculate the mean ΔP by:

$$\text{mean } \Delta P = \frac{\sum_{i=1}^{n} 4v_n^2}{n}$$

1.10   Limitations of Doppler Measurements

In order to have accurate and reliable Doppler measurements, operators need to be aware of two main limitations in Doppler measurement: (1) Doppler angle error in velocity measurement and (2) the assumptions of the modified Bernoulli equation (MBE) in pressure gradient measurements.

1.10.1   Doppler Angle Error

To obtain accurate velocity measurements, the ultrasound beam needs to be parallel to the flow, i.e. Doppler angle = $0°$. The velocity will be underestimated when the Doppler angle deviates from $0°$ (Fig. 1.10). The operator should minimise

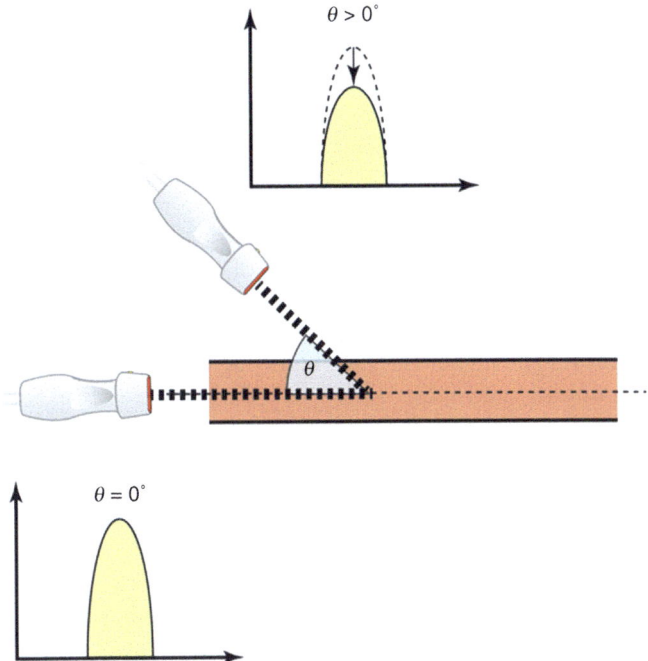

FIGURE 1.10 Effects of Doppler angle (θ) on blood flow velocity

this angle to less than 20°, which corresponds to <10% under-estimation of velocity.

1.10.2   Assumptions of SBE

The SBE assumes that:

1. Blood flow is laminar.
2. Blood flow is non-pulsatile.
3. There is no resistance to blood flow.
4. The density of blood is constant.

Violation of any of the above assumptions leads to inaccurate estimation (underestimation) of the pressure gradient.

Bernoulli's assumptions are mostly valid when blood is flowing across a small orifice, such as stenosis and regurgitation, and is centrally directed into the distal chamber.

1.11   Aliasing

Aliasing only occurs in PW Doppler where ultrasound is transmitted in pulses. The rapidity of the pulses transmitted (or pulse repetition frequency (PRF)) (see above) determines the maximal blood flow velocity (v_{max}) the PW Doppler can measure. The higher the PRF is, the higher is the v_{max}. In most ultrasound machines, the v_{max} is usually between 1.5 and 1.7 m/s.

1.11.1   Appearance of Aliasing in PW Doppler

When the blood flow velocity is higher than the v_{max}, such as a regurgitant or stenotic jet, **aliasing** occurs. Aliasing is characterised by the inability of the screen to show the high-velocity region (above v_{max}), and that region is 'cut' and 'paste' above the baseline if blood is flowing away from the transducer (or below the baseline if blood is flowing towards the transducer). This is known as the 'wrap-around' phenomenon (Fig. 1.11).

Practical Tips: Correction of Aliasing

Aliasing can be corrected by one or more of the following manoeuvres:

1. Increasing the velocity scale
2. Shifting the baseline
3. Increasing PRF (use high PRF mode)
4. Reducing transducer frequency

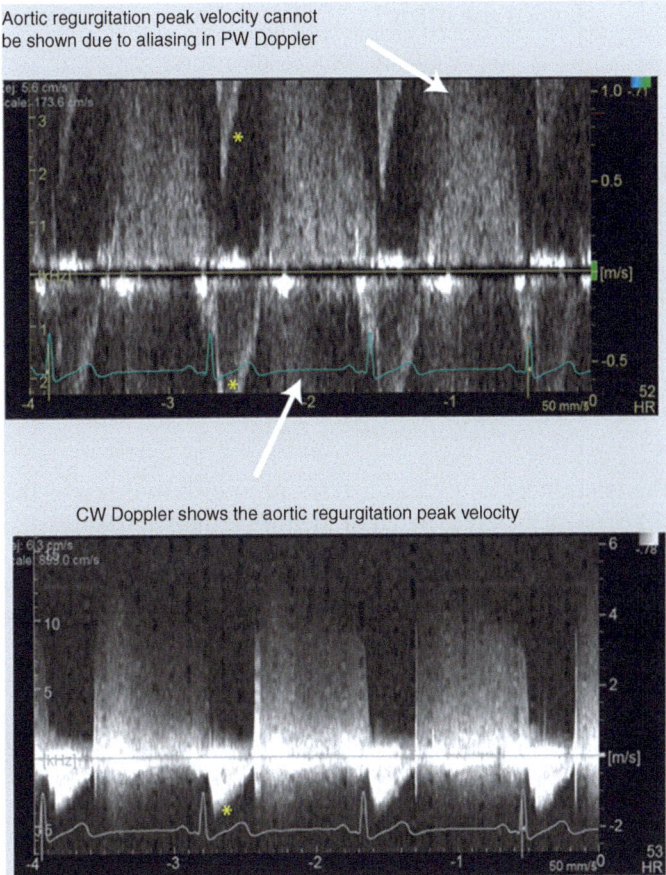

FIGURE 1.11 Aliasing and 'wrap-around' phenomenon. Upper diagram shows a PW Doppler spectrum in the left ventricular outflow tract. The spectrum consists of both LVOT flow (∗) and aortic regurgitation (AR) (arrow). However, aliasing (wrap around) is seen with the high-velocity AR Doppler spectrum continue from below. Similarly, the LVOT flow was also discontinued at the bottom but was displayed at the top. Lower diagram shows the spectrum obtained using CW Doppler

1.12   Color Doppler

Color Doppler, also known as **color flow mapping**, is used to visualise blood flow in echocardiography and vascular ultrasound. Using different colours and saturation, the direction and velocity of blood flow can be appreciated on the screen. Color Doppler uses multiple PW Doppler sample volumes to gather flow (velocity) information over an area, as defined by the **color box**. The velocities from each sample volumes are then represented by different colors and are shown on the screen.

1.12.1   Direction of Blood Flow

The transducer is used as a reference point to describe the direction of blood flow. Flow is flowing either towards the transducer or away from the transducer. Although any two colors can be chosen to represent the two directions, the widely accepted convention is to use blue and red—**B**lue is flowing **A**way from the transducer and **R**ed is **T**owards the transducer (**BART**) (Fig. 1.12).

1.12.2   Velocity of Blood Flow

Blood flow velocity is denoted by the color saturation, with lighter color representing faster velocity. Hence, for blood flowing away from the transducer, one may see different shades of blue, some lighter in color and some deeper in color.

1.12.3   Aliasing in High Velocity Flows

As pulsed Doppler is used in colour Doppler, it is also subject to the aliasing phenomenon when blood flow velocity exceeds v_{max}. In a simple two colour (red-blue) flow map, 'wrap-

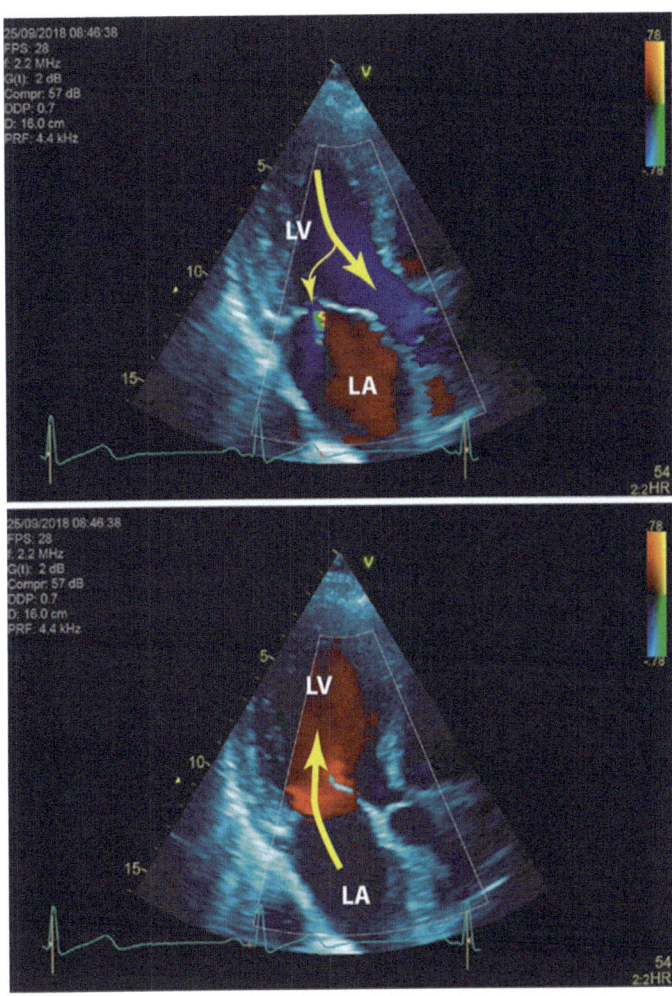

FIGURE 1.12 Color Doppler. Upper: blood exiting left ventricle (LV) during systole (thick yellow arrow). Flow appears blue as blood is flowing away from the transducer. Mild mitral regurgitation is also present (small arrow). Lower: during diastole, blood is flowing from left atrium (LA) from LV and appears red

around' is shown as the opposite colour. Where a variance colour flow map is used (most common setting), aliasing is presented as a different color (e.g. green). When flow is turbulent, a mosaic color is shown.

1.13   Tissue Doppler Imaging

1.13.1   Tissue Doppler Velocity

Cardiac function can be estimated by measuring the velocity of the myocardium. Myocardial velocity can be measured using PW Doppler by placing the sample gate at the AV valve annulus. For RV function, the sample volume is placed at the tricuspid annulus, and for LV function, the sample volume is placed at the mitral annulus, commonly at the medial (septal) and lateral aspect.

1.13.2   Components of Tissue Doppler Velocity

Normally, three main waves can be identified (Fig. 1.13):

- **S** wave: the systolic velocity of ventricular contraction
- **E′** wave: the early diastolic velocity of ventricular relaxation
- **A′** wave: the late diastolic velocity due to atrial contraction

Quite often, an isovolumic contraction (IC) or isovolumic relaxation (IR) waves can also be seen.

Systolic and diastolic dysfunction is associated with a reduction in S and E′ wave, respectively.

1.13.3   Limitations of TDI

- Angle dependence
- Misplacement of sample gate location: velocity will be underestimated if the sample volume is placed below the AV valves
- Yielding of global regional information only and inability to give specific segmental wall information

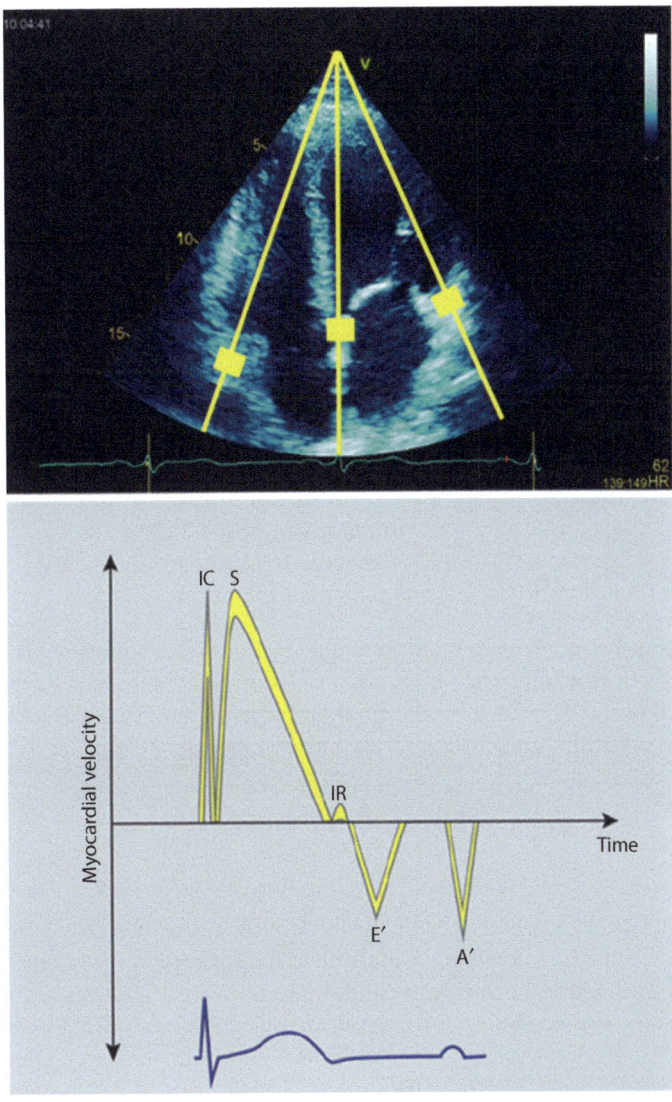

FIGURE 1.13 Tissue Doppler velocity. Upper: tissue Doppler sample volume is placed at the mitral or tricuspid annulus. Lower: components of typical tissue Doppler waveforms in a normal (healthy) patient

1.14   Ventricular Strain Measurement

Strain is a measure of **deformation**. In echocardiography, strain is often used for studying ventricular wall deformation.

1.14.1   Deformation of the Ventricle

When the ventricles contract and relax, the myocardium changes shape (deforms). For example, a healthy myocardium becomes thicker and shorter in systole, and thinner and longer in diastole. A diseased myocardium may fail to change shape (akinetic); hence there is no deformation or zero strain. Strain is commonly used to study ventricular systolic function.

1.14.2   Strain

Systolic strain is defined as the degree a myocardium **shortens** or **thickens** when compared to its original (starting) state. Hence, if L_1 and L_0 is the final and starting length (or thickness) of the myocardium, respectively, then

$$\text{Strain} = \frac{L_1 - L_0}{L_0} \times 100\%$$

For myocardial shortening, strain is negative because L_1 is less than L_0. For myocardial thickening where L_1 is greater than L_0, strain is a positive number.

1.14.3   Types of Strain

There are three different types of ventricular strain measurements (Fig. 1.14):

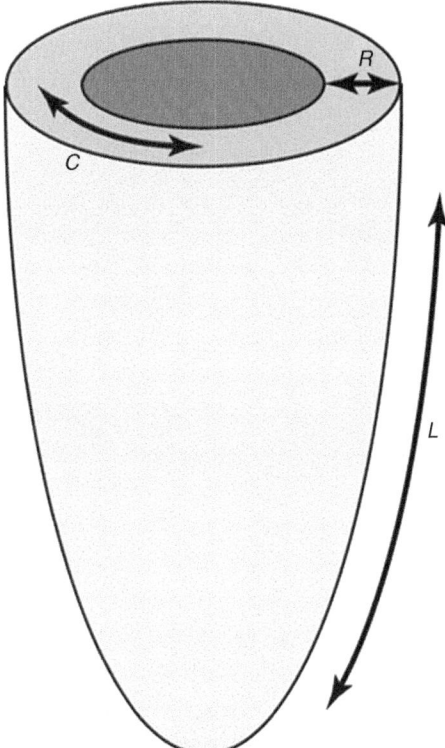

FIGURE 1.14 Different types of strains. Schematic diagram showing circumferential (C), radial (R) and longitudinal (L) strains of the left ventricle

1. **Longitudinal strain**, which measures the longitudinal contraction, hence shortening, of the ventricle.
2. **Radial strain**, which measures the systolic thickening of the ventricular wall; this is usually measured in the cross-sectional (short-axis) view of the ventricle.
3. **Circumferential strain**, which measures the systolic shortening of ventricle in the cross-section (short axis) view.

Further, strain can be **segmental** or **global**. Segmental strain yields regional wall motion information. Global strain gives the overall strain of the whole ventricle.

Part I
TEE and TTE Views

Chapter 2
Transthoracic Echocardiography: Views and Measurements

Stephen J. Huang

2.1 Challenges in TTE Examination

The main challenges in performing TTE are the presence of bones and air-filled lung blocking the ultrasound beam pathway to the heart due to acoustic impedance mismatch (see Chap. 1). To perform TTE, one must avoid these structures to access the heart. Fortunately, two windows are available for accessing the heart in TTE (Fig. 2.1):

1. The left parasternal window formed by the rib space and the costomediastinal recess
2. The apical window provided by the rib space and the costodiaphragmatic recess at the left lower lung margin

The liver also provides an excellent acoustic window for accessing the heart and inferior vena cava via the subcostal window (Fig. 2.1).

S. J. Huang (✉)
Intensive Care Unit, Nepean Hospital, University of Sydney
Nepean Clinical School, Sydney, NSW, Australia
e-mail: Stephen.huang@sydney.edu.au

© Springer Nature Switzerland AG 2020
M. Slama (ed.), *Echocardiography in ICU*,
https://doi.org/10.1007/978-3-030-32219-9_2

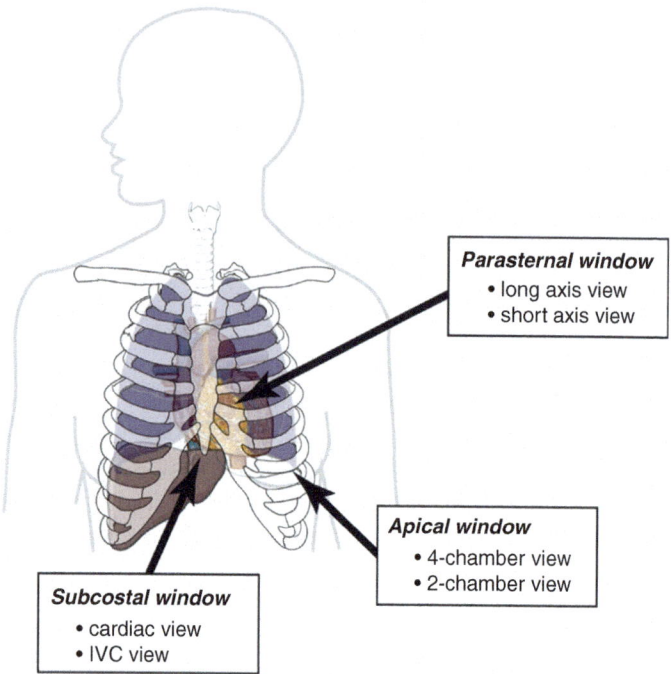

FIGURE 2.1 The three windows and six views of TTE. There are three windows and six views in TTE. The parasternal window takes advantage of the intercostal space and the costomediastinal recess. The apical window, where the probe is placed over the apex of the heart, takes advantage of the intercostal space and costodiaphragmatic recess. The subcostal window makes use of the liver as an acoustic window

2.2   Patient Preparation and Probe Selection

Patient details (e.g., name, height and weight) should be entered into the machine before the start of the TTE examination, and the electrocardiographic (ECG) cable should be connected. If possible, patients should lie in the left lateral recumbent position with the left arm raised and rested on the pillow. This position widens the rib space and costomediastinal recess; hence it helps to access the parasternal windows (see below).

While this is not a rule, experienced intensive care sonographers prefer to perform the examination on a patient's left side by holding the probe using the left hand. It offers several advantages:

- The sonographer can see the patients and interact (communicate) with them face to face.
- Workplace injury is reduced by not having to extend the right arm over the patient if the examination is performed on the patient's left side. This is especially important in big patients.

A phase-array cardiac probe should be used for examination because of its small footprint and frequency range. The small footprint allows one to fit the probe between rib spaces, hence avoiding rib shadows that block the view of the heart. These probes commonly have a frequency range of 2–4 MHz, which provides a good compromise of image resolution and penetration.

2.3   Acoustic Windows

There are three windows and six views in a routine TTE for intensive care patients (Fig. 2.1):

- Parasternal window:
    - Parasternal long axis (PL) view
    - Parasternal short axis (PS) view

- Apical window:
    - Apical 4 chamber (A4) view
    - Apical 2 chamber (A2) view

- Subcostal window:

    - Subcostal cardiac (SC) view
    - Subcostal inferior vena cava view (SIVC) view

The procedure of TTE follows the above windows and view sequence:

PL → PS → A4 → A2 → SC → SIVC

2.3.1   The Parasternal Long Axis (PL) View

The PL view is usually the starting point of the TTE. The acoustic window is the intercostal space in the costomediastinal recess (Figs. 2.1 and 2.2). The probe is usually placed between the third and the fifth intercostal space on the left sternal border, although more superior or inferior probe positions are not uncommon in intensive care patients.

The PL view is the longitudinal section of the left ventricle (LV). To obtain the longitudinal view, the pointer of probe should be pointing around the right shoulder of the patient. Slight probe rotation (clockwise or counter-clockwise) is usually needed to ensure that the ultrasound plane is along the central longitudinal axis of the LV (Fig. 2.3).

Various important structures can be visualized in this view: aorta (Ao), left atrium (LA), LV, and right ventricle (RV) (outflow tract). Interrogation of aortic and mitral valve structure and function can also be done. The PL view is also the first view to pick up pericardial effusion.

2.3.1.1   Measurements

The dimensions of the LV, LA, and aorta Ao are usually measured in this view. Motion mode (M-mode) is the preferred method for measurements. Certain technical points should be taken into account when performing M-mode measurements:

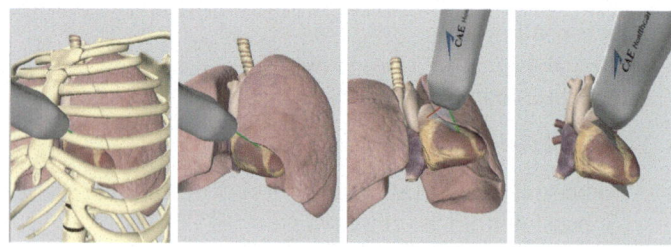

FIGURE 2.2 The TTE parasternal window. The probe is placed between the third and the fifth intercostal space in the costomediastinal recess

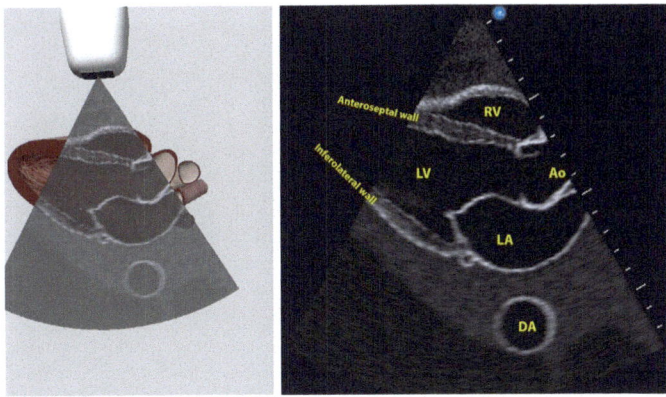

FIGURE 2.3 The parasternal long-axis (PL) view. Right: the PL view is the longitudinal section of the LV; hence, the ideal ultrasound plane is along the central axis of the LV. Left: PL view is displayed on screen. *Ao* aorta, *DA* descending aorta, *LA* left atrium, *LV* left ventricle, *RV* right ventricle

1. The operator should make sure that the largest chamber size is obtained by tilting the probe to and fro.
2. The operator should also ensure that the M-mode cursor is orthogonal to the chamber's long axis; otherwise, the dimension can be overestimated.
3. For LV measurement, the cursor should be placed at the mitral leaflet tip during early diastole. For Ao-LA measurement, the cursor should be placed at the aortic sinuses (Fig. 2.4).

The following measurements can be obtained:

- LV M-mode
  - LV end-diastolic antero-septal wall thickness
  - LV end-diastolic diameter
  - LV end-diastolic infero-lateral wall thickness

- Aorta-LA M-mode
  - Ao end-diastolic diameter
  - LA end-systolic diameter

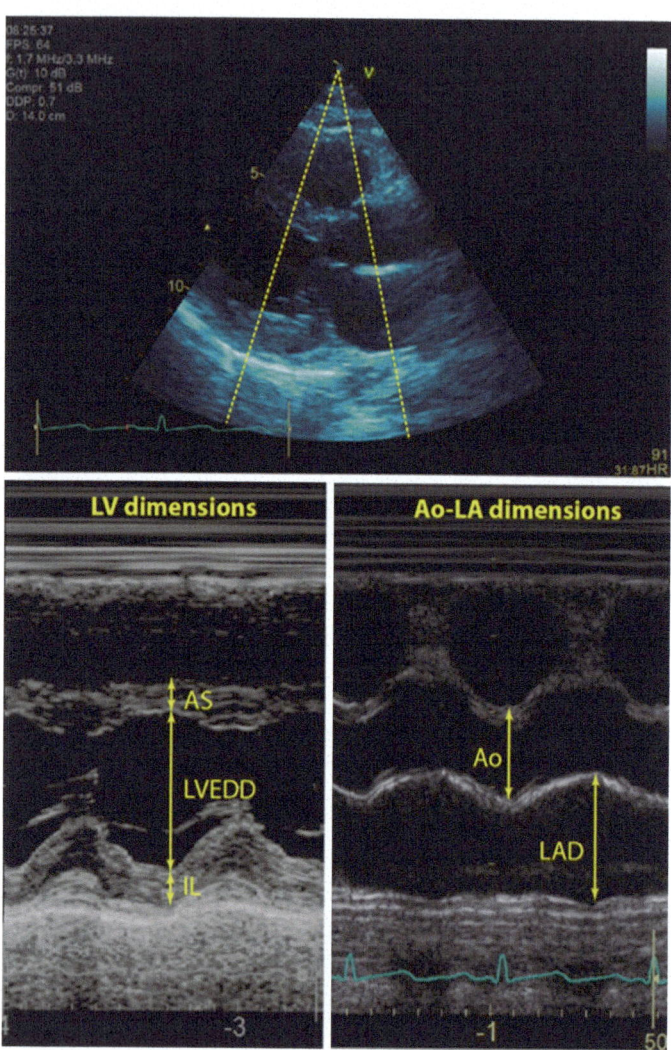

FIGURE 2.4 M-modes at the PL view. Two M-mode cursors are shown (top), one for the LV dimension and the other for Ao-LA dimension measurements. LV dimension M-mode is shown in the lower left, whereas Ao-LA dimension M-mode is shown in the lower right. *Ao* aorta, *AS* anteroseptal wall, *IL* inferolateral wall, *LAD* LA diameter, *LVEDD* LV end-diastolic diameter

Leading-edge-to-leading-edge method is used for M-mode measurements. If it is impossible to obtain a perpendicular angle with the cursor, anatomical M-mode, if available, can be used. Otherwise, measurements can be made using 2D images. Normal range is shown in Table 2.1.

TABLE 2.1 Chamber dimensions reference values [1, 2]

Parameter	Reference range[a] Female	Male
LV end-diastolic diameter, mm	38–53	42–59
LV end-diastolic diameter (indexed), mm/m^2	24–32	22–31
LV end-diastolic volume (biplane), ml	46–106	62–150
LV end-diastolic volume (indexed), ml/m^2	29–61	34–74
Interventricular septum thickness, mm	6–9	6–10
Inferolateral (posterior) wall thickness, mm	6–9	6–10
LA area, cm^2	≤20	≤20
LA area index, cm^2/m^2	59–127	59–119
LA volume, ml	22–52	18–58
LA volume index, ml/m^2	16–34	16–34
RV basal diameter, mm	24–42	24–42
RV mid-cavity diameter, mm	20–35	20–35
RA area, cm^2	≤20	≤20
RA volume index, ml/m^2	16–34	16–34
Annulus (LV outflow tract), mm	19–27	20–32
Sinuses of Valsalva, mm	24–36	28–40
Sinotubular junction, mm	20–32	23–35
Proximal ascending aorta, mm	19–35	22–38

[a]Reference range = mean ± 2 SD

Two-dimensional measurements are particularly useful in situations where the cardiac axis is tilted (angulated) or when the translational artifact is severe for the M-mode. High frame rates are required to ensure that 2D measurements are made at the right phase of the cardiac cycle.

2.3.2   The Parasternal Short Axis (PS) View

PS view provides the cross-sections of the heart. To obtain the view, the probe is rotated 90° clockwise from the PL position. The pointer should be pointing around the left shoulder. Four levels (or sections) of PS view can be obtained by tilting and/ or moving the probe longitudinally (Fig. 2.5). PS examination starts from the supraventricular (aortic level) to the apex of the LV:

- Aortic valve view
- The base of the LV or mitral valve view
- Mid-ventricular view
- Apical view

Various structures can be identified in these views (Fig. 2.6). The biggest advantage of PS view is that clear visualization of the aorta, tricuspid valve, pulmonary valve, and various LV wall segments can be obtained.

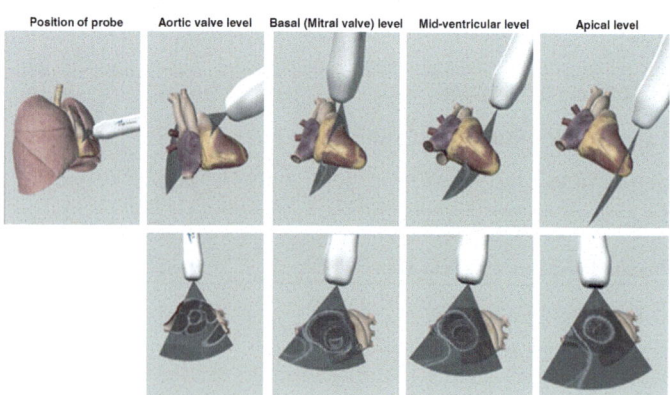

FIGURE 2.5 The parasternal short-axis (PS) view

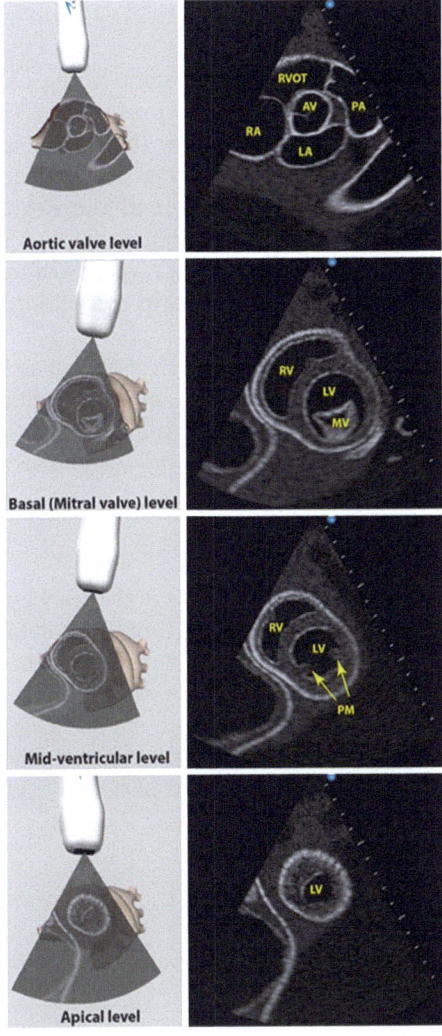

FIGURE 2.6 Various structures seen in the PS view. The aortic level is characterized by the presence of aortic valve at the center, being surrounded by right ventricular outflow tract (RVOT), pulmonary artery (PA), left and right atria (LA and RA) clockwise, respectively. Mitral valve (MV) can be seen in the basal level. Papillary muscle (PM) is the "marker" of the mid-ventricle. The disappearance of papillary muscle and the systolic obliteration of the LV are the signs of reaching the apical level

2.3.3   The Apical-4-Chamber (A4) View

The probe is placed at the apical region of the LV in the A4 view, with the pointer directed posteriorly (Fig. 2.7). Although the acoustic window is provided by the costodiaphragmatic recess, the probe's position can vary greatly depending on the position of the patient, lung size and the degree of lung hyperinflation, and other factors. For example, the probe is more medial when the patient is in supine position, whereas a more lateral placement is needed in the left lateral recumbent position.

In the A4 view, one can see the LV, RV, and atria (LA and RA) (Fig. 2.8), and it is one of the most important views to measure chamber sizes (areas and volumes). The whole of the LV inferoseptal and anterolateral walls can be visualized.

2.3.3.1   Measurements

Various measurements can be made in the A4 view, including LV and LA volumes, RV diameter, and RA volumes. LV volumes are usually measured using Simpson's method, whereas LA and RA volumes can be measured using either the Simpson's method or the area-length method (Fig. 2.9).

RV volumes are not measured due to its noncylindrical crescentic shape. Hence, RV diameter is reported instead (Fig. 2.10).

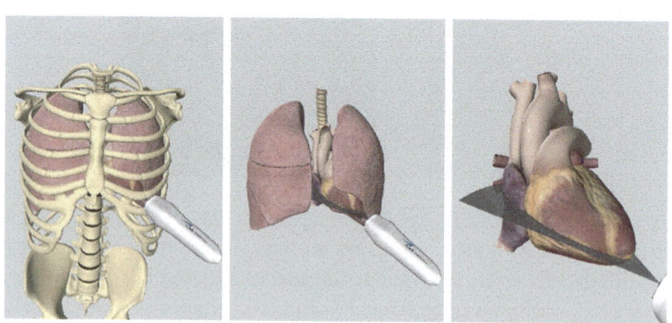

FIGURE 2.7 Probe position for the apical-4-chamber (A4) view

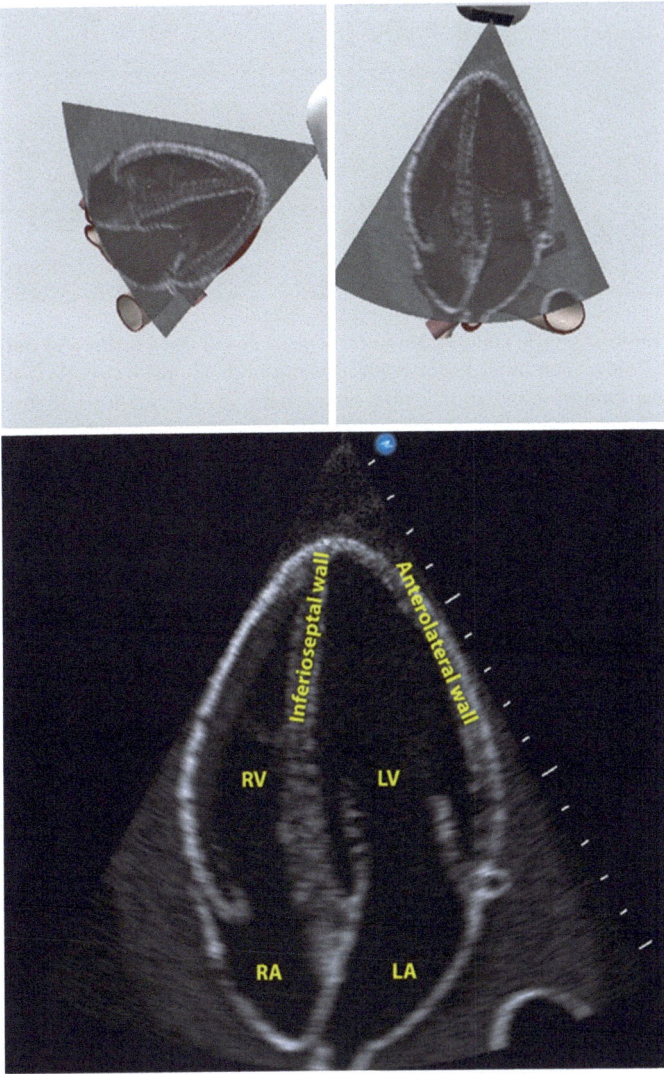

FIGURE 2.8 The apical-4-chamber (A4) view. The diagrams show the correlation of the ultrasound plane (top left and right) and A4 view shown on the display (lower). Top left and right, view from left infero-lateral side

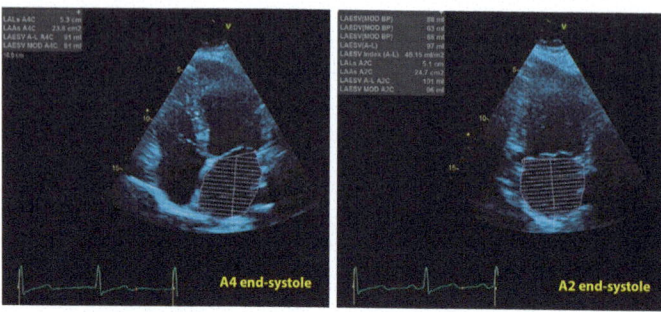

FIGURE 2.9 LA volume measurements. LA volumes in the A4 and A2 views (biplane) are measured using both Simpson's method of disc summation (MOD) and area-length (A-L) methods in this example. The volumes obtained from the two views should be averaged. Note that the length of the LA (LALs), measured from the mitral annulus plane to the superior border of the LA, in both views are approximately the same (5.3 cm vs. 5.1 cm)

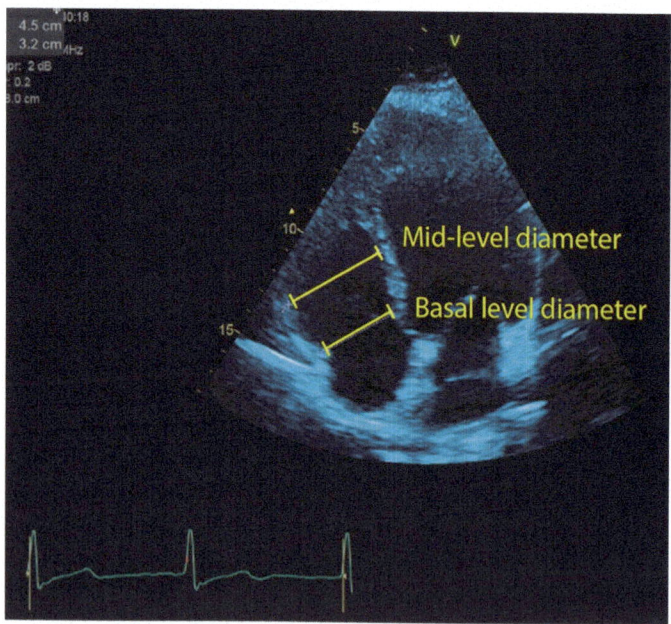

FIGURE 2.10 RV diameter measurements in 2D image

2.3.4 The Apical-2-Chamber (A2) View

The A2 view is obtained by rotating the transducer in the A4 position by approximately 60° counterclockwise (Fig. 2.11). This view allows the visualization of the LV and LA only, hence the name "2-chamber." The anterior and inferior walls are captured in this view (Fig. 2.11).

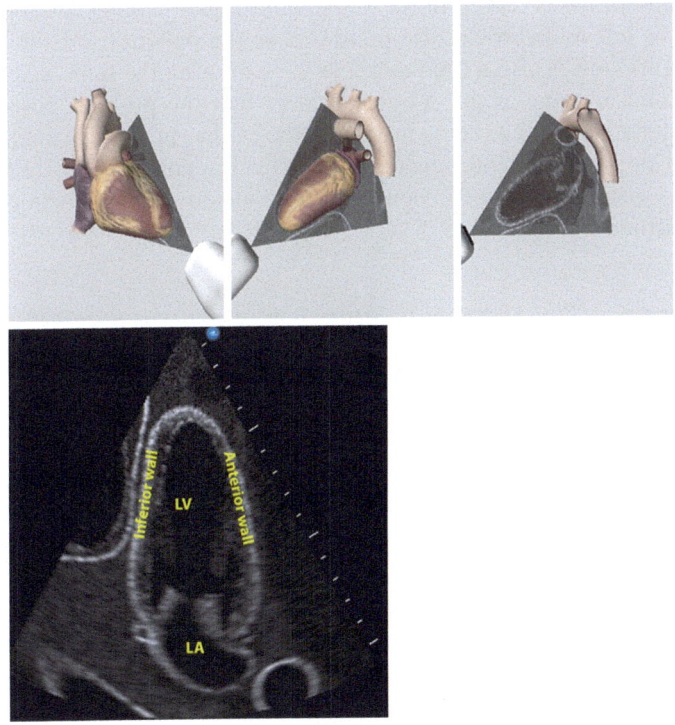

FIGURE 2.11 RV diameter measurements in 2D image. Ultrasound plane of A2 view as seen from the anterior (top left) and left lateral (top middle). A sectioned view from the left lateral side is shown in the top right, with the 2D image shown below

2.3.4.1   Measurements

LV and LA volumes are also measured in this view for biplane measurements (Fig. 2.9).

2.3.5   *The Subcostal Cardiac View*

The probe is placed in the subxiphoid region aiming toward the left mid-clavicle. The pointer is to the patient's left side. This view is also a four-chamber view offering the same anatomical plane as the A4 view, except that the probe is positioned in the RV region instead of the cardiac apex (Fig. 2.12). This provides a full view of the RV, which is normally difficult to visualize in the A4 view due to rib-shadow and refraction artifacts (Fig. 2.13).

2.3.6   *The Subcostal Inferior Vena Cava (SIVC) view*

To obtain the SIVC view, the probe is rotated approximately 90° counterclockwise from the SC view and point posteriorly. The pointer should be at the 12 o'clock position and should be tilted slightly to the patient's right side (off midline) to get a full longitudinal inferior vena cava (IVC) view (Fig. 2.14).

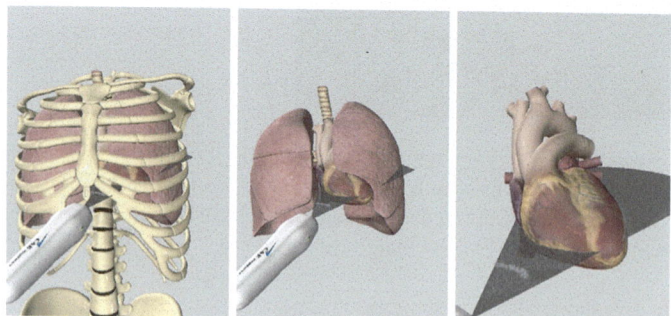

Figure 2.12 The subcostal cardiac view

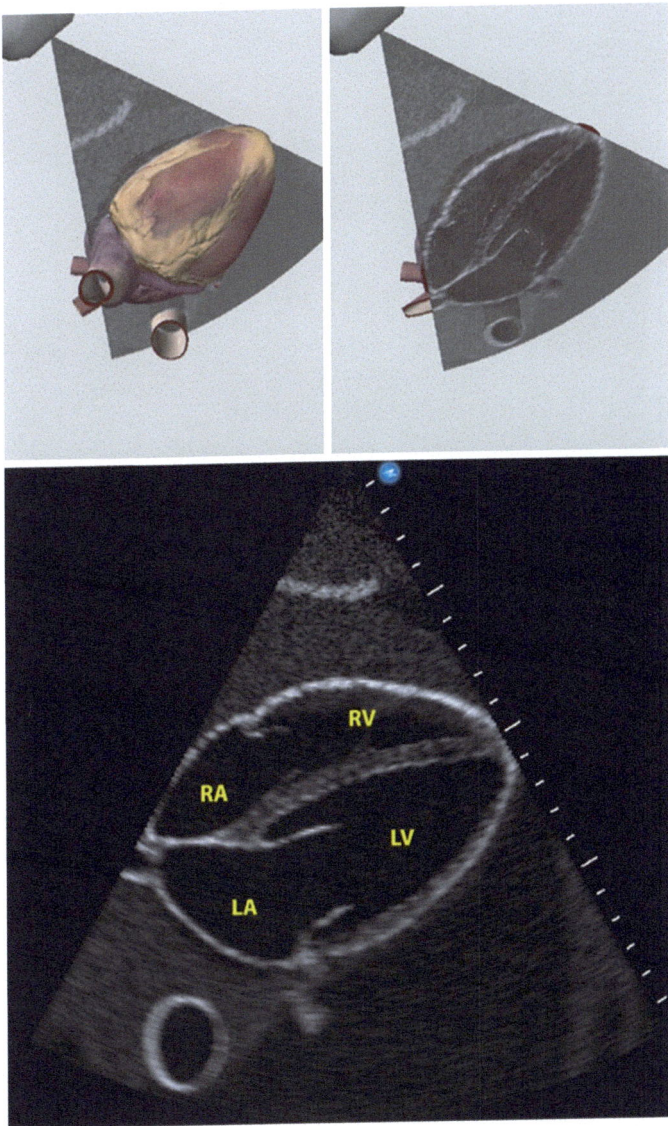

Figure 2.13 The 4 chamber view in the subcostal cardiac view. Ultrasound plane as seen from postero-inferior angle

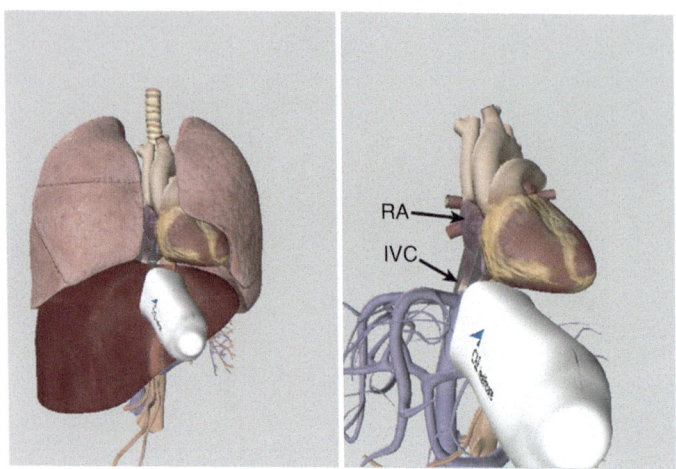

FIGURE 2.14 Probe position in the subcostal IVC (SIVC) view

One should ensure that the vessel drains directly into the RA, is nonpulsatile and does not taper distally (Fig. 2.15).

2.3.6.1 Measurements

IVC is used for fluid status (preload and fluid responsiveness) assessments (see Chap. 9). These assessments rely on accurate measurements of IVC diameters during inspiration and expiration. IVC diameter is normally obtained from M-mode, although 2D measurements are also used, especially in situations where translational artifacts from respiration are present (Fig. 2.16); Table 2.1 provides all normal values.

2.4 Summary

A bedside TTE for intensive care patients consists of three windows and six views. In the order of sequence of a routine study, these views are PL, PS, A4, A2, SC, and SIVC. These views complement each other and should be used to confirm or rule out abnormal findings (e.g., wall motion defects or

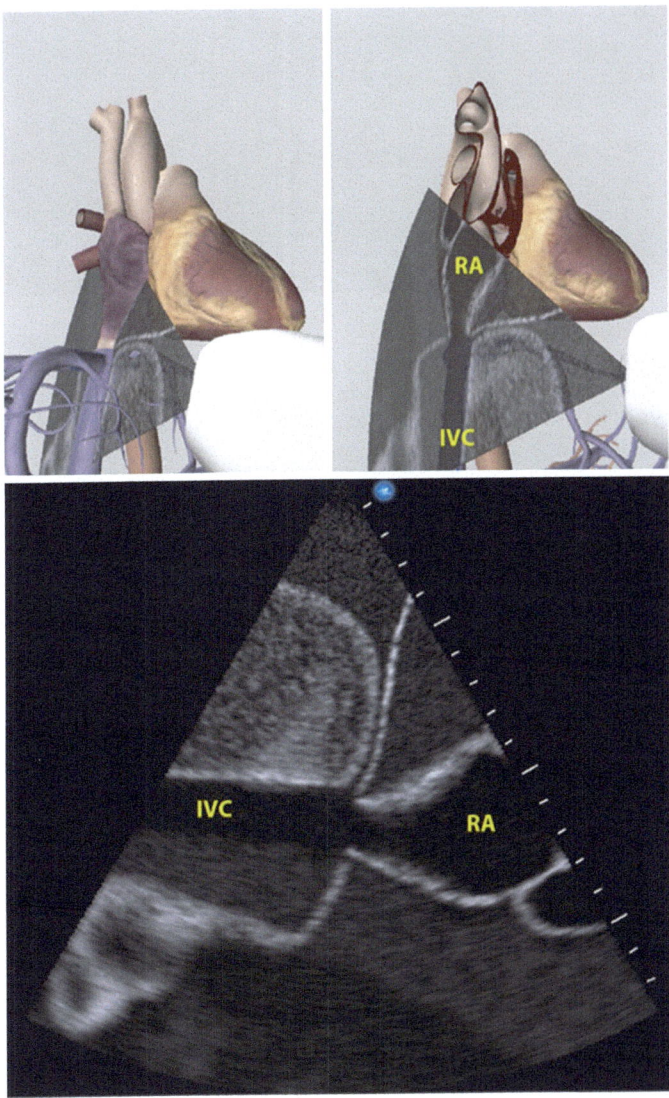

FIGURE 2.15 The subcostal IVC view. Note the IVC drains directly into the RA

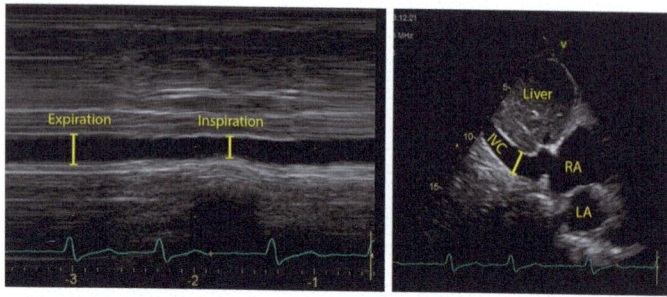

FIGURE 2.16 Measurement of IVC. IVC diameters at expiration and inspiration are usually measured using M-mode (left, yellow bars). Two-dimensional image can also be used for the measurement of IVC diameters (right, yellow bar). Patient shown here was breathing spontaneously

presence of thrombus) in any one view. Measurements of chamber size or dimensions are usually done by M-mode in virtue of its high frame rate, but 2D measurements are also sometimes used.

Acknowledgment   Many 3D figures were obtained using CAE Vimedix cardiac ultrasound simulators. The author would like to thank CAE Healthcare (https://www.caehealthcare.com) for allowing the use of the 3D figures.

Multiple Choice Questions

1. Which of the following is NOT a determinant of TTE image quality?

    A. Patient's body size
    B. Patient's heart size
    C. Types of probe
    D. Patient's position
    Answer: B

2. Which of the following is false?

    A. Phased array probe is best for TTE because it got the smallest footprint.
    B. Measurements, except for IVC, are best done at end expiration.

  C. Patients need to be in the left recumbent position when having TTE.
  D. None of the above.
  Answer: C

3. Which of the following views is not part of a usual TTE examination?

  A. Parasternal views
  B. Apical views
  C. Subcostal views
  D. Right parasternal view
  Answer: D

4. Which of the following about parasternal window is false?

  A. It provides a longitudinal view.
  B. It is the only window that provides a proper transverse view.
  C. Pericardial effusion can be seen in this window.
  D. All of the above.
  Answer: D

5. Which of the following is a challenge in TTE?

  A. Displaying ECG on the screen.
  B. Obtaining parasternal view in patients with larger pericardial effusion.
  C. Obtaining apical view in patients with larger pericardial effusion.
  D. Obtaining parasternal view in patients with hyperinflated lungs.
  Answer: D

References

1. Lang RM, Badano LP, Mor-Avi V, Afilalo J, Armstrong A, Ernande L, et al. Recommendations for cardiac chamber quantification by echocardiography in adults: an update from the American Society of Echocardiography and the European Association of Cardiovascular Imaging. J Am Soc Echocardiogr. 2015;28(1):1–39.

2. Rudski LG, Lai WW, Afilalo J, Hua L, Handschumacher MD, Chandrasekaran K, et al. Guidelines for the echocardiographic assessment of the right heart in adults: a report from the American Society of Echocardiography endorsed by the European Association of Echocardiography, a registered branch of the European Society of Cardiology, and the Canadian Society of Echocardiography. J Am Soc Echocardiogr. 2010;23(7):685–713.

Chapter 3
Transoesophageal Echo Views and Measurements

Sam Orde

Transoesphageal echo (TEE or TOE) can be used for diagnostic and haemodynamic monitoring. It is an invasive technique and therefore requires adequate training, suitable equipment and monitoring, as well as analysis of benefits vs. risks (please see Chap. 5).

3.1 Tips and Tricks

- Use systematic approach to scanning, but be opportunistic if a suitable window becomes available (e.g. left atrial appendage).
- Avoid excessive probe anteflexion and retroflexion when in the oesophagus.

Electronic Supplementary Material   The online version of this chapter (https://doi.org/10.1007/978-3-030-32219-9_3) contains supplementary material, which is available to authorized users.

S. Orde (✉)
Nepean Hospital, Sydney, NSW, Australia

© Springer Nature Switzerland AG 2020
M. Slama (ed.), *Echocardiography in ICU*,
https://doi.org/10.1007/978-3-030-32219-9_3

- If you see an abnormality in one plane, review it in another.
- Don't force probe advancement if obstruction is felt.
- Doppler angles are often not ideal; try different views if possible.
- If you get lost, go back to 0° and find a standard view.

3.2 Probe Insertion

Pearls	• Follow the contour of the soft and hard palate when inserting into the oropharynx by gentle retroflexion then anteflexion.
	• Keep gentle constant pressure to get past the larynx (ask patient to 'swallow' if they are sufficiently awake).
	• Have patient centred in bed with your advancing hand in midline when inserting to ensure that the probe is advancing in the midline.
	• Consider laryngoscopy in intubated patients.
	• Use jaw thrust and flex the head when inserting into the oesophagus.
	• Use gentle retroflexion at the larynx to advance into the oesophagus.
Pitfalls	• Ensure probe 'lock' is **off** when inserting.
	• Have adequate oropharynx topical localisation to minimise sedation requirements if patient is awake.
	• Have an assistant hold endotracheal tube in intubated patient during probe insertion/withdrawal.

3.3 Probe Movements

Advance ↔ withdraw	Fig. 3.1a
Omniplane rotation: 0° ↔ 180°	Fig. 3.1b
Probe rotation: left ↔ right	Fig. 3.1c
Anteflexion ↔ retroflexion	Fig. 3.1d

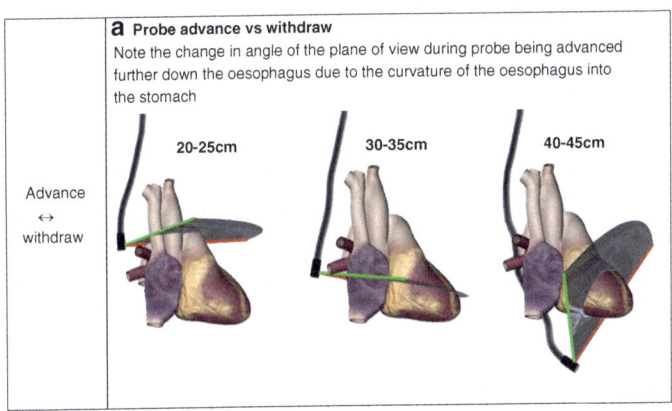

FIGURE 3.1A Probe advance vs. withdraw. Note the change in the angle of the plane of view when the probe is being advanced further down the oesophagus due to the curvature of the oesophagus into the stomach

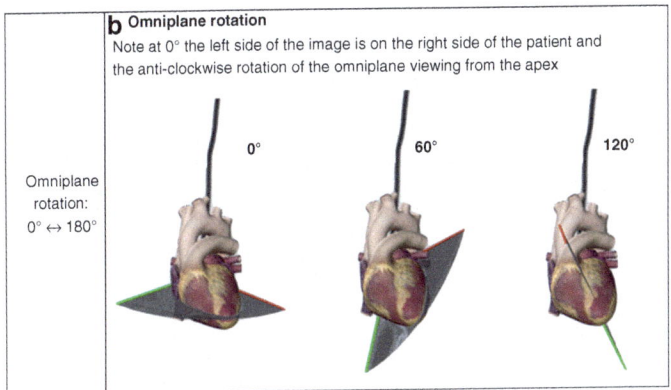

FIGURE 3.1B Omniplane rotation: Note at 0° the left side of the image is the right side of the patient. Increasing the omniplane angle causes anti-clockwise rotation (looking up at heart from apex)

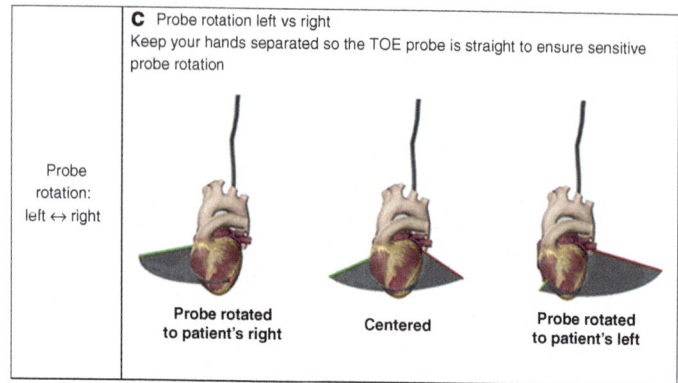

FIGURE 3.1C   Probe rotation left vs. right. Keep your hands separated so that the TOE probe is straight to ensure sensitive probe rotation

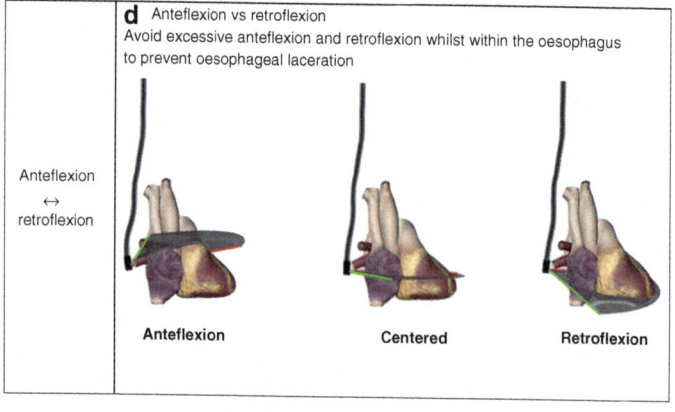

FIGURE 3.1D Anteflexion vs. retroflexion. Avoid excessive anteflexion and retroflexion whilst within the oesophagus to prevent oesophageal laceration

3.4   Procedure

A TEE should be performed systematically to ensure that structures and pathology are not missed. Several structured sequences are possible. We present one method that starts in the deep gastric view, then the probe is removed, reviewing structures along the way. Finally, the probe is re-advanced then slowly removed again to review the aorta.

Tip: Minimise anteflexion/retroflexion movements whilst in the oesophagus.

3.4.1   Deep Gastric View

View	Omiplane angle	Probe depth (from teeth)	Probe position	Chambers/ structures	Assessment
Deep gastric view	0°	~40–45 cm	Full anteflexion	Left ventricle (LV) LV outflow tract (LVOT) Aortic valve	LV size and function Aortic valve flow LVOT flow respiratory variation

Deep gastric view enables one of the best Doppler angles to interrogate LVOT and aortic valve flows.

Tip: Push the probe into 50 cm until the probe tip is deep in the stomach (no images visible). Perform full anteflexion, then pull the probe back *slowly* until the tip is held against the apex. NB: avoid pulling the probe into the oesophagus in full anteflexion as damage may occur (Fig. 3.2).

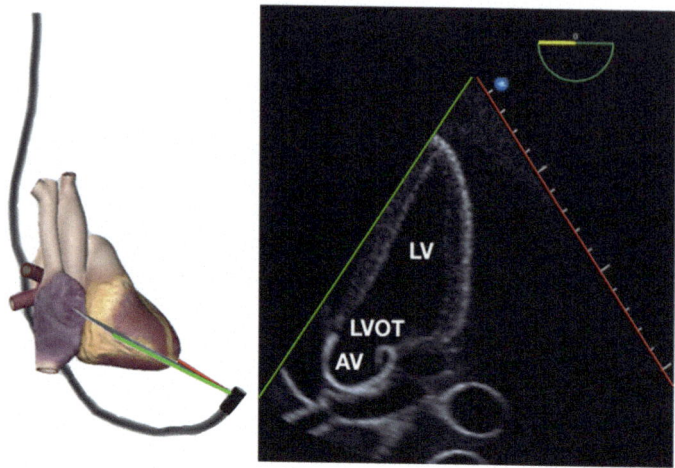

FIGURE 3.2 Deep gastric view: full anteflexion with probe in stomach (~45cm). NB: ensure you are deep in the stomach before anteflexing to avoid damaging the lower oesophagus

3.4.2 Transgastric Views

View	Omniplane angle	Probe depth (from teeth)	Probe position	Chambers/structures	Assessment
Transgastric short-axis view (Fig. 3.3a)	0°	~35–40 cm	Neutral	Left ventricle (apical, mid-papillary level and mitral valve level) Right ventricle	Left ventricle size and function Regional wall motion Right ventricle size and function
Transgastric two-chamber view (Fig. 3.3b)	90°	~35–40 cm	Neutral	Left ventricle	Left ventricle size and function Regional wall motion

View	Omniplane angle	Probe depth (from teeth)	Probe position	Chambers/ structures	Assessment
Transgastric right ventricle inflow view (Fig. 3.3c)	90°	~35–40 cm	Neutral Directed right	Right ventricle	Right ventricle size and function Tricuspid valve flows
Transgastric long-axis view (Fig. 3.3d)	120°	~35–40 cm	Neutral	Left ventricle (LV) LV outflow tract (LVOT) Aortic valve	LV size and function Aortic valve flow LVOT flow respiratory variation

Tip: If the view is suboptimal, use **gentle** anteflexion to improve contact with the oesophagus.

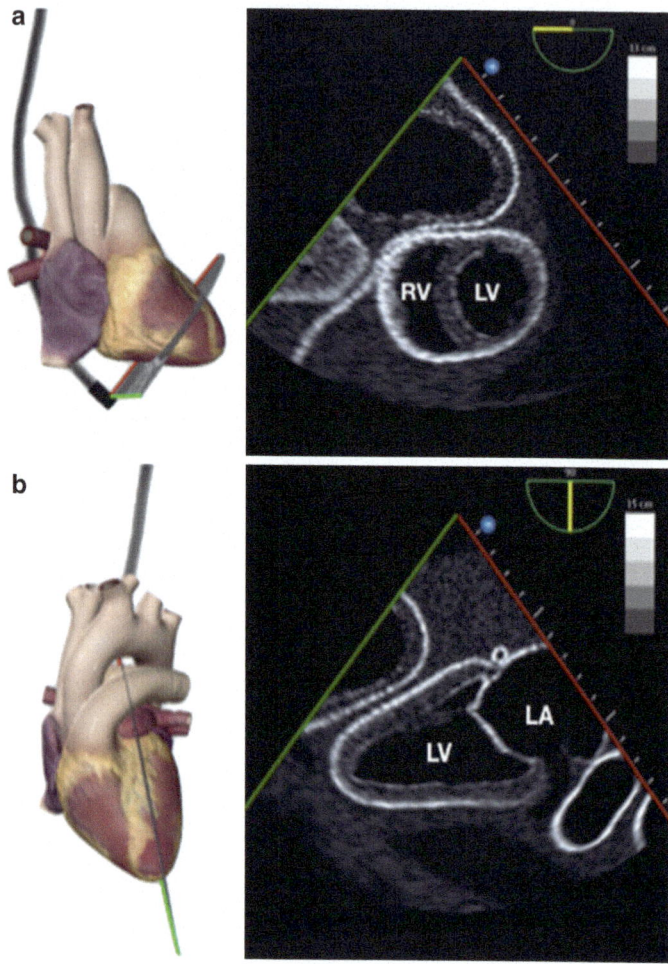

FIGURE 3.3 Transgastric views: (**a**) Short axis view, (**b**) two chamber view, (**c**) right ventricle inflow view, (**d**) long axis view

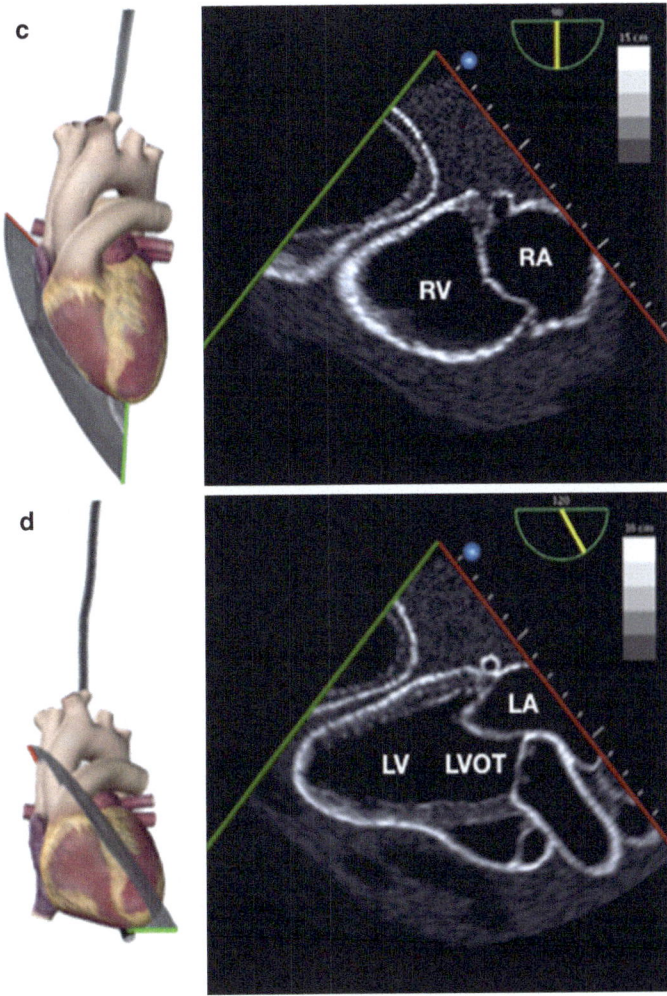

FIGURE 3.3 (continued)

3.4.3   Mid-Oesophageal Views

View	Omniplane angle	Probe depth (from teeth)	Probe position	Chambers/structures	Assessment
Mid-oesophageal four-chamber view (Fig. 3.4a)	0°	~30–35 cm	Retroflexed	Left ventricle Left atrium Right ventricle Right atrium	Left ventricle size and function Regional wall motion Right ventricle size and function Atria size
Mid-oesophageal mitral commissural or two-chamber view[a] (Fig. 3.4b)	60–90°	~30–35 cm	Retroflexed	Left ventricle Left atrium	Left ventricle size and function Regional wall motion
Mid-oesophageal long-axis view (Fig. 3.4c)	120°	~30–35 cm	Retroflexed	Left ventricle Left ventricle outflow tract Aortic valve Right ventricle	Left ventricle size and function Left ventricle outflow tract

View	Angle	Depth	Probe position	Structures	Doppler/assessment
Mid-oesophageal left atrial appendage view (Fig. 3.4d)	110°	~30–35 cm	Retroflexed	Left ventricle, Left atrium, Left atrial appendage	Left atrial appendage flows[a]
Mid-oesophageal aortic short-axis view (Fig. 3.4e)	30°	~30 cm	Neutral	Aortic valve, Left atrium, Right atrium, Right ventricle	Tricuspid valve flows, Interatrial septal defects
Mid-oesophageal bicaval view (Fig. 3.4f)	110°	~30 cm	Neutral, Directed right	Left atrium, Right atrium, Superior vena cava, Inferior vena cava	Interatrial septal defects, Superior vena cava respiratory variation[b]

[a] Left atrial appendage flows <0.4 m/s suggest decreased flow

[b] Superior vena cava respiratory variation >36% in a fully mechanically ventilated patient suggest fluid responsiveness

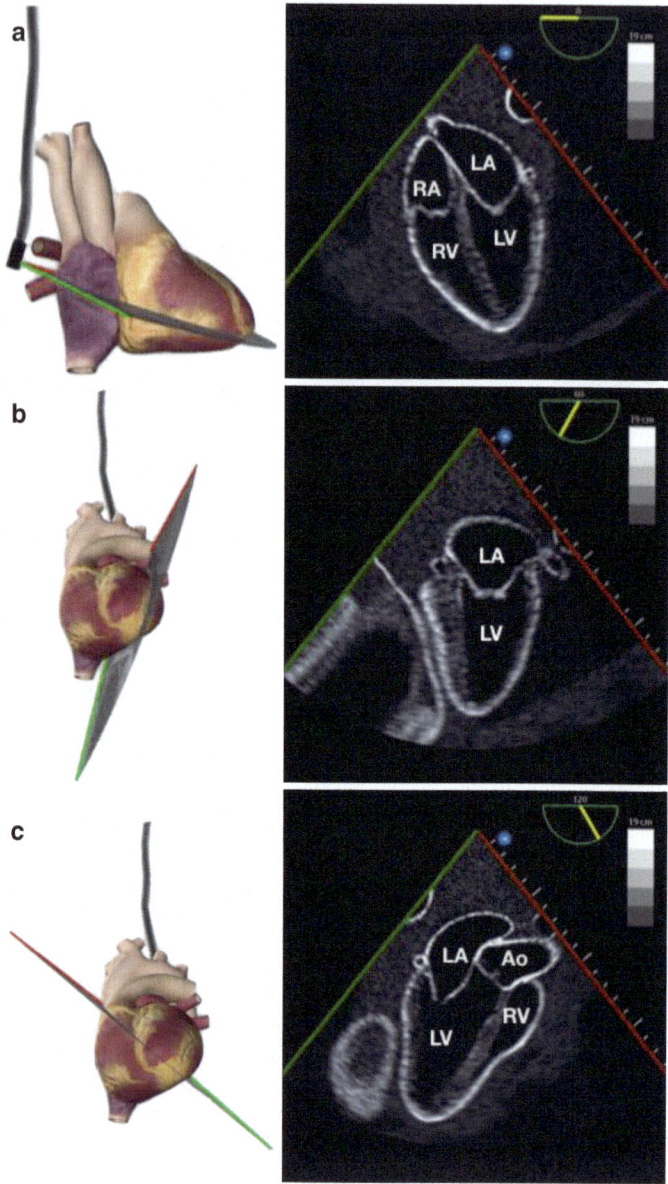

FIGURE 3.4 Mid-oesophageal views: (**a**) four chamber view, (**b**) mitral commissural view, (**c**) long axis view, (**d**) left atrial appendage view, (**e**) aortic valve short axis view, (**f**) bicaval view

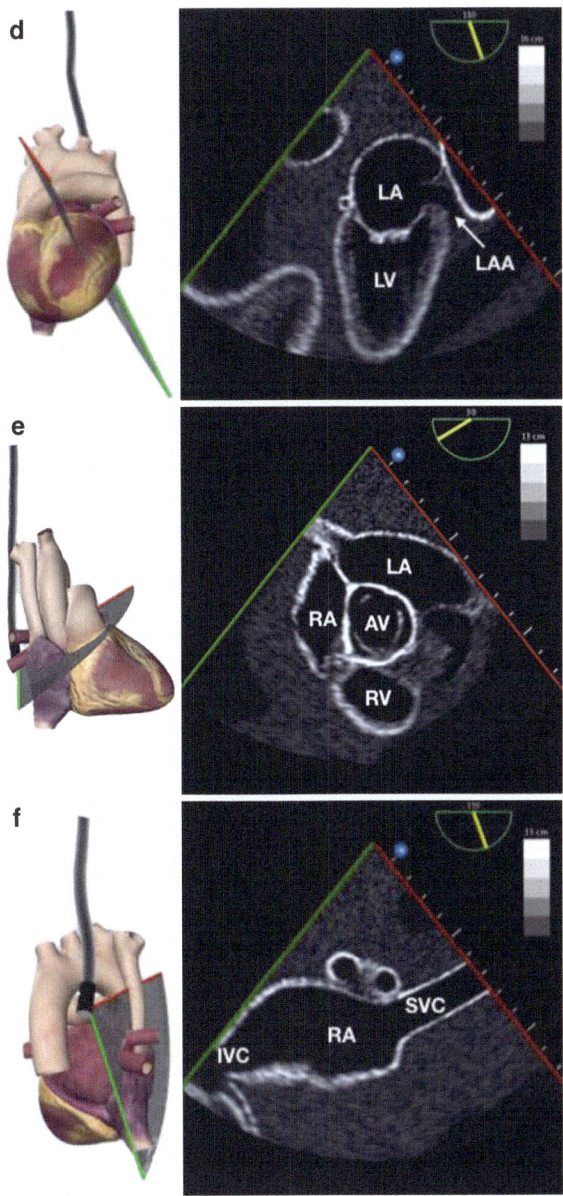

FIGURE 3.4 FIGURE 3.4 (continued)

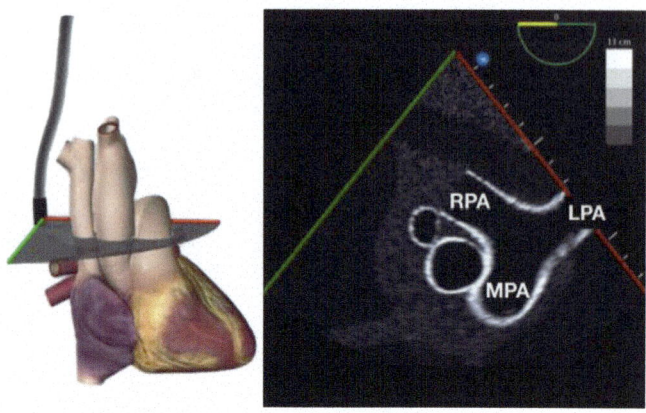

FIGURE 3.5 High oesophageal view

3.4.4   High Oesophageal View

View	Omiplane angle	Probe depth (from teeth)	Probe position	Chambers/ structures	Assessment
Pulmonary artery view (Fig. 3.5)	0°	~20–25 cm	Neutral	Pulmonary artery	Right and left pulmonary artery Main pulmonary artery trunk

3.4.5   Aorta Views

View	Omiplane angle	Probe depth (from teeth)	Probe position	Chambers/ structures	Assessment
Aorta views (Fig. 3.6a, b)	0° and 90°	~25–45 cm	Neutral Directed posteriorly	Aorta	Aorta size Dissection flaps Presence of atheroma[a]

[a]Mild atheroma: 1–2 mm, moderate: 2–4 mm, severe: >4 mm

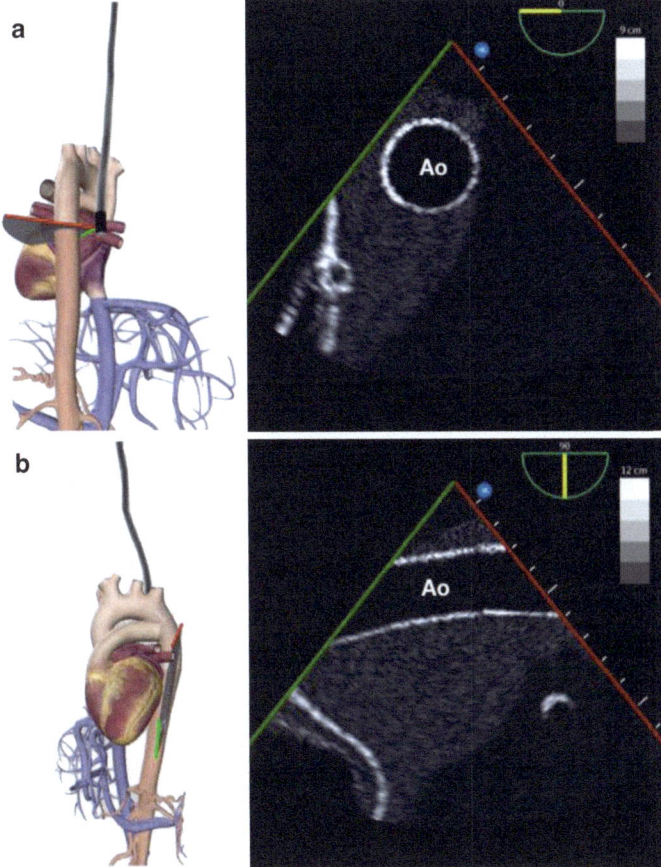

FIGURE 3.6 Aorta views: (**a**) short axis view, (**b**) long axis view

Multiple Choice Questions

1. Which of the following TEE views is the best for assessing aortic valve flows?

    A. Mid-oesophageal four-chamber view
    B. Deep gastric view
    C. Transgastric short-axis view
    D. Mid-oesophageal commissural view

E. Bicaval view
Answer: B

2 Which TEE view can be used to assess the anterior left
ventricle wall?

A. Mid-oesophageal four-chamber view
B, Bicaval view
C. Mid-oesophageal short-axis view
D. Mid-oesophageal commissural view
E. Bicaval view
Answer: D

3. What structure is the arrow pointing at?

A. Left atrium
B. Left ventricle
C. Left atrial appendage

1. Left atrium
2. Left ventricle
3. Left atrial appendage
4. Pulmonary valve
5. Left ventricle outflow tract

D. Pulmonary valve
E. Left ventricle outflow tract
Answer: C

4. Which of the following is the best method for assessing
fluid responsiveness with echo in a fully mechanically ventilated patient?

A. Superior vena cava respiratory variation greater than
36%
B. LVOT Vmax respiratory variation less than 20%

C. Aortic valve VTI respiratory variation less than 20%
D. Inferior vena cava collapse with insufflation greater than 50%
E. Left ventricle fractional area change in short-axis view greater than 50%

Answer: A

6. A patient with a DVT has a recent stroke and you're performing a TEE to assess a patent foramen ovale. Which of the following views is best to assess this?

A. Mid-oesophageal four-chamber view
B. Transgastric short-axis view
C. Mid-oesophageal long-axis view
D. Deep gastric view
E. Bicaval view

Answer: E

Chapter 4
Artifacts

Philippe Vignon

Artifacts refer to any image that fails to correlate directly with an underlying actual anatomical structure or tissue. They result from errors in the acoustic presentation of the examined organ, which are caused by technical limitations or anatomical factors. Importantly, artifacts may lead to diagnostic errors with potentially devastating therapeutic consequences. Numerous artifacts have been described when using two-dimensional [1] and also three-dimensional echocardiography [2].

4.1 Artifacts Related to Reflection and/or Refraction

These artifacts are the most commonly encountered. Linear artifacts are related to the reverberation of the ultrasound wave between two strong reflectors, one of them being potentially the transducer itself [3]. When located within the aortic lumen, linear artifacts may be misinterpreted as actual flaps in the setting of patients assessed using transesophageal

P. Vignon (✉)
Medical-Surgical Intensive Care Unit, Dupuytren Teaching Hospital, Limoges, France

Inserm CIC-P 1435, Dupuytren Teaching Hospital, Limoges, France
e-mail: philippe.vignon@unilim.fr

© Springer Nature Switzerland AG 2020   65
M. Slama (ed.), *Echocardiography in ICU*,
https://doi.org/10.1007/978-3-030-32219-9_4

echocardiography for a suspected aortic dissection or disruption [4]. This misleading image can be observed within the ascending aorta whenever its size exceeds that of the anatomical structure interposed between the aorta and the transducer [3]. This accounts for its high prevalence (26%) and illustrates the risk of misinterpretation with a flap in a patient presenting with a dilated aorta [4] (Fig. 4.1).

Mirror artifacts are also commonly observed. The pericardium (transthoracic echocardiography) or the pleura (transesophageal echocardiography) may constitute strong acoustic interfaces for ultrasound propagation that result in a duplicated image of the heart or the descending aorta [1]. In the latter case, the true aortic wall should not be interpreted as an intimal flap separating two distinct channels consistent with associated aortic dissection (Fig. 4.2).

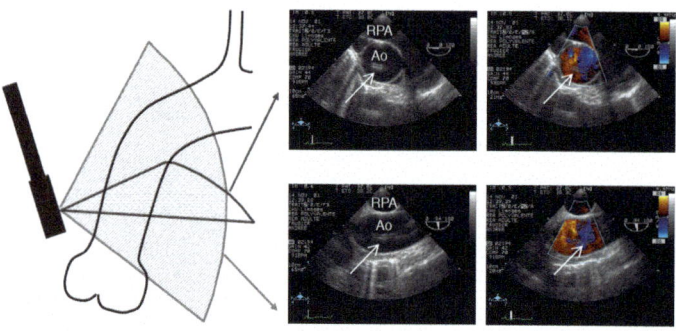

FIGURE 4.1 Linear artifact in the ascending aorta depicted by transesophageal echocardiography in a ventilated patient presenting with an acute aortic syndrome. In both the transversal (upper panels) and the longitudinal planes (lower panels), a thick linear image that moves parallel to the aortic walls in real time and is almost horizontal (left panels, arrow) is evidenced. Color Doppler mapping depicts a normal linear flow over imposed on this linear image in both views, with similar blood flow velocities on both sides of the linear image, but no aliasing consistent with blood flow turbulence (right panels, arrow). Abbreviations: *Ao* ascending aorta, *RPA* right pulmonary artery

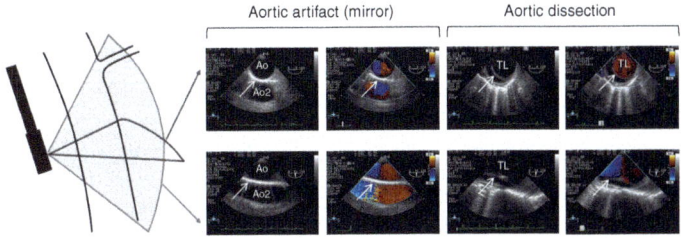

FIGURE 4.2 Transesophageal echocardiography performed in two patients for a suspected acute disease of the descending thoracic aorta. In the first patient, the presence of a mirror artifact of the descending thoracic aorta results from the presence of a strong acoustic interface (left air-filled lung and intravascular blood; left panels, arrow) and is observed in both the transverse (upper panels) and longitudinal views (lower panels). Normal blood flow pattern evidenced using color Doppler mapping is also duplicated, both images being separated by the normal aortic wall (middle left panels, arrow). The second patient sustained a type B aortic dissection, as evidenced by the presence of an actual intimal flap (middle-right panels, arrow), which separated a circulating true lumen from a non-circulating false channel during color flow mapping (right panels, arrow). Abbreviations: *Ao* descending thoracic aorta, *Ao2* mirror image of the descending aorta, *TL* true lumen

4.2 Other Artifacts

Various other artifacts have been described using two-dimensional echocardiography [1]. Acoustic shadowing is frequently related to calcified structures or prosthetic elements located within the heart. The use of transesophageal echocardiography may be particularly useful to provide adequate visualization of anatomical structures hidden by acoustic shadowing. Side-lobe artifacts are "arc-like" linear images that may be created within the ascending aorta and misinterpreted as intimal flaps. Near-field clutter is located in the apical region of the left ventricle and should not be interpreted as a mural thrombus [1]. Three-dimensional echocardiography generates also artifacts, including images compatible with an intraluminal thrombus or vegetation [5].

4.3   Facts or Artifacts?

> **Box 4.1 The Presence of at Least Three Criteria Among the Previous Is Specific of a Linear Artifact Within the Ascending Aorta**
>
> 1. Displacement of the linear image parallel to aortic walls.
> 2. Similar blood flow velocities on both sides of the linear image using color Doppler mapping.
> 3. Thickness of the linear image >2.5 mm.
> 4. Angle between the linear image and the aortic wall >85° (nearly horizontal image) [4]. M-mode is helpful in precisely depicting the motion of the intra-aortic image during the cardiac cycle [6]. The linear artifact moves parallel to the aortic walls, whereas the intimal flap follows the pressure gradient between the two lumens of the aortic dissection during the cardiac cycle (Fig. 4.3).

As a general rule, alternative imaging planes or even alternative approaches (e.g., computed tomography) should be routinely used to best differentiate artifacts from true abnormalities that must be systematically confirmed in distinct echocardiographic views. The influence of gains on the questionable image favors the diagnosis of artifacts [1]. The use of color Doppler mapping is helpful when depicting normal laminar blood flow over imposed on the abnormal image (Fig. 4.1) but may still be misleading in the presence of mirror artifacts (Fig. 4.2). Finally, alternative imaging modality may be required to confidently exclude the diagnosis of artifact and to best guide patient's management [5].

Linear artifact   Aortic dissection

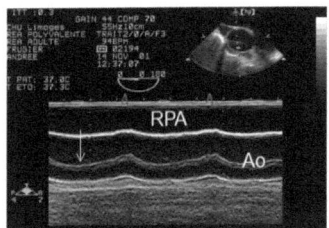 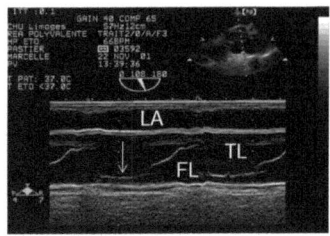

FIGURE 4.3 Use of transesophageal echocardiographic M-mode to differentiate a linear artifact of the ascending aorta from a true intimal flap of a type A acute aortic dissection. The linear artifact appears as a thick image with a displacement remaining strictly parallel to the aortic walls during the cardiac cycle (left panel, arrow). In contrast, the intimal flap is thinner and follows the pressure gradient between the two delimited channels of the aortic dissection, the true lumen expanding during systole (right panel, arrow). Abbreviations: *Ao* ascending aorta, *RPA* right pulmonary artery, *LA* left atrium, *TL* true lumen, *FL* false lumen

Multiple Choice Questions

1. The diagnostic criteria used to identify a linear artifact in the ascending aorta when assessing a patient using transesophageal echocardiography are:

   A. A thin freely mobile linear image
   B. A thick linear image with a displacement parallel to aortic walls during the cardiac cycle
   C. The presence of similar blood flow velocities on both sides of the linear image during color Doppler mapping
   D. The nearly horizontal position of the linear image
   E. A variable angle between the linear image and the aortic wall

   Answers: B, C, D

2. Potential means to avoid or identify artifacts associate:
   A. Use of alternative imaging planes
   B. Modifications of gains
   C. Use of color Doppler mapping with appropriate Nyquist limit
   D. Preferable use of transthoracic echocardiography
   E. Preferable use of transesophageal echocardiography
   Answers: A, B, C

References

1. Bertrand PB, Levine RA, Isselbacher EM, Vandervoort PM. Fact or Artifact in Two-Dimensional Echocardiography: Avoiding Misdiagnosis and Missed Diagnosis. J Am Soc Echocardiogr. 2016;29(5):381–91.
2. Faletra FF, Ramamurthi A, Dequarti MC, Leo LA, Moccetti T, Pandian N. Artifacts in three-dimensional transesophageal echocardiography. J Am Soc Echocardiogr. 2014;27(5):453–62.
3. Appelbe AF, Walker PG, Yeoh JK, Bonitatibus A, Yoganathan AP, Martin RP. Clinical significance and origin of artifacts in transesophageal echocardiography of the thoracic aorta. J Am Coll Cardiol. 1993;21(3):754–60.
4. Vignon P, Spencer KT, Rambaud G, Preux PM, Krauss D, Balasia B, Lang RM. Differential transesophageal echocardiographic diagnosis between linear artifacts and intraluminal flap of aortic dissection or disruption. Chest. 2001;119(6):1778–90.
5. Goudelin M, Hernandez Padilla AC, Gonzalez C, Vignon P. Real-time three-dimensional transesophageal echocardiography fails to discriminate between infectious vegetation and artifact. Intensive Care Med. 2018;44(6):992–4.
6. Evangelista A, Garcia-del-Castillo H, Gonzalez-Alujas T, Dominguez-Oronoz R, Salas A, Permanyer-Miralda G, Soler-Soler J. Diagnosis of ascending aortic dissection by transesophageal echocardiography: utility of M-mode in recognizing artifacts. J Am Coll Cardiol. 1996;27(1):102–7.

Part II
Echocardiography in ICU

Chapter 5
Echocardiography in the ICU: When to Use It?

Philippe Vignon

Critical care echocardiography (CCE) is performed and interpreted by the front-line intensivist at the bedside to establish diagnoses and help guide the management of severely ill patients with cardiopulmonary compromise. Basic-level CCE is a prerequisite training for every intensivists. It relies on a goal-directed examination using preferentially transthoracic echocardiography (TTE) to identify specific findings and to answer a limited number of straightforward clinical questions. Advanced-level CCE is an optional component of the training of ICU physicians. It allows performing a comprehensive hemodynamic assessment using adapted quantitative parameters obtained with transesophageal echocardiography (TEE) if required.

> CCE is the preferred modality to initially evaluate the type of shock as opposed to more invasive techniques.

P. Vignon (✉)
Medical-Surgical Intensive Care Unit, Dupuytren Teaching Hospital, Limoges, France

Inserm CIC-P 1435, Dupuytren Teaching Hospital, Limoges, France
e-mail: philippe.vignon@unilim.fr

© Springer Nature Switzerland AG 2020
M. Slama (ed.), *Echocardiography in ICU*,
https://doi.org/10.1007/978-3-030-32219-9_5

Indications for performing advanced CCE are numerous and may be influenced by specific ICU recruitments such as cardiac surgery or trauma patients (Tables 5.1 and 5.2).

TABLE 5.1 Respective characteristics of basic and advanced critical care echocardiography (CCE)

Basic CCE	Advanced CCE
Goal: goal-oriented examination to answer a limited number of clinical questions	*Goal*: comprehensive examination to be self-sufficient in conducting hemodynamic assessment
Principle: favors specificity over sensitivity	*Principle*: adapts the diagnostic workup to the clinical scenario and therapeutic interventions
Means: qualitative assessment based on two-dimensional imaging and color Doppler mapping[a]	*Means*: quantitative assessment based on all available echocardiographic modalities[b]
Diagnostic field: narrow • Overt hypovolemia • Left ventricular failure • Right ventricular failure • Tamponade • Acute massive left-sided valvular regurgitation • Mechanism of cardiac arrest • Heterogeneous contraction patterns	*Diagnostic field*: broad • Circulatory failure/shock of any origin: leading mechanisms, underlying cardiac diseases (cardiomyopathy, valvulopathy, valvular prosthetic dysfunction), complicated cardiac surgery, circulatory assistance • Cardiac arrest: potential (reversible) cause, postresuscitation circulatory failure • Acute respiratory failure of any origin: left-sided filling pressure, level of pulmonary artery hypertension, consequences on right ventricular function of lung disease and ventilator settings, anatomical shunts • Specific clinical settings: infective endocarditis, systemic embolism, acute aortic syndrome, cardiovascular trauma, brain dead donor, guidance of invasive procedures…

Table 5.1 (continued)

Basic CCE	Advanced CCE
Modality of use: • Punctually (diagnosis) • Serially (efficacy and tolerance of therapy)	*Modality of use*: • Punctually (diagnosis) • Hemodynamic monitoring (clinically driven)
Certification: not required	*Certification*: recommended
Target: every intensivists (required training)	*Target*: optional component of the training

[a]Mainly with transthoracic echocardiography
[b]Including transesophageal echocardiography

TABLE 5.2 Main indications of advanced critical care echocardiography (CCE)

Diagnostic scope of advanced CCE

Circulatory failure/shock: cardiac output, underlying myocardial or valvular disease, monitoring efficacy, and tolerance of therapeutic interventions
• Tamponade (pericardial, loculated or not, extrapericardial)
• Fluid responsiveness (irrespective of ventilation mode, cardiac rhythm, and abdominal pressure)
• Left ventricular systolic function (including longitudinal myofiber shortening)
• Right ventricular systolic function (right ventricular failure and ventricular interdependency)
• Vasoplegia (diagnosis of elimination)
• Circulatory assistance (related complications, weaning)
• Postcardiac surgery circulatory failure (any of the above mechanism, surgical complications)

Cardiac arrest:
• During resuscitation: tamponade, massive pulmonary embolism, cardiac standstill vs. fibrillation
• After resuscitation: fluid responsiveness, left or right ventricular dysfunction, vasoplegia, and potentially associated cardiomyopathy[a]

(continued)

Table 5.2 (continued)

Diagnostic scope of advanced CCE

Acute respiratory failure[b]: monitoring efficacy and tolerance of therapeutic interventions
- Quantitative assessment of left ventricular filling pressure
- Identification and severity assessment of potential underlying myocardial or valvular disease
- Determination of the level of pulmonary artery hypertension (acute on chronic vs. acute)
- Right ventricular systolic function (right ventricular failure and ventricular interdependency)
- Intracardiac or intrapulmonary anatomical shunt (severity for participation in hypoxemia)
- Identification of "dynamic events" (i.e., increase of left filling pressure, worsening of a mitral or aortic regurgitation, dynamic left ventricular outflow tract obstruction, right ventricular failure) during abrupt changes of cardiac loading conditions (e.g., spontaneous breathing trial, changes of ventilator settings), or body position (platypnea-orthodeoxia syndrome)

Specific clinical settings:
- Infective endocarditis: identification of vegetations (assess risk of embolization), abscesses, and valve perforation; severity assessment of resulting valvular regurgitation
- Systemic embolism: identification of cardiac or aortic sources of systemic embolization (e.g., thrombus, tumor, atheromatous debris), depiction of patent foramen ovale (paradoxical embolism[c])
- Acute aortic syndrome: identify aortic dissection, intramural hematoma, penetrating atheromatous ulcer, (false-)aneurysm formation, and extravasation signs (hemopericardium, hemomediastinum, hemothorax, hemoperitoneum); identify mirror and linear artifacts as potential false-positive diagnoses
- Cardiovascular trauma: identify blunt aortic and cardiac trauma, determine the depth of aortic injury (related to the risk of lethal adventitial rupture) and its suitability for endovascular repair (anatomical extension, complexity of injury, location relative to the take-off of the sub-clavian artery, pseudo-coarctation syndrome, size of the false-aneurysm formation and of the vessel)
- Brain dead donor: guide resuscitation (fluid responsiveness, left or right ventricular dysfunction, vasoplegia), determine suitability for heart donation
- Guide invasive procedures: pericardocentesis, internal pacing, placement of venous cannula of circulatory assistance/extracorporeal membrane oxygenation

[a]Same as circulatory failure/shock
[b]Combine CCE with thoracic ultrasound for best diagnostic capacity
[c]Combine CCE with venous ultrasound for diagnosing deep venous thrombosis

When compared to "blind" hemodynamic assessment based on thermodilution techniques (i.e., pulmonary artery catheter, transpulmonary thermodilution), advanced CCE provides direct quantitative information on central hemodynamics, respective right and left ventricular function, and potential underlying cardiac disease. Accordingly, CCE is superior to thermodilution-based techniques to identify false positive results of pulse pressure variation to predict fluid responsiveness when related to acute right ventricular failure; combine several dynamic indices, including passive leg raising, to best predict cardiac response to fluid loading; ascribe a low flow state to the most failing ventricle and accurately identify right ventricular failure; determine how left ventricular stroke volume is generated (contractility versus enlarged cavity), and depict severe valvulopathy or prosthetic valve dysfunction, left ventricular outflow tract obstruction, or markedly low flow states, which may interfere with a thermodilution-based hemodynamic assessment.

Advanced CCE encompasses both TTE and TEE assessments, according to their respective advantages and limitations. TEE must be performed in patients with suspected localized tamponade, valve prosthesis dysfunction, infective endocarditis, acute aortic diseases, systemic or pulmonary embolism, or patent foramen ovale or for the guidance of certain invasive procedure (e.g., right heart cannulation, aortic stenting) since it has a greater diagnostic accuracy than surface echocardiography in these clinical settings (Table 5.3).

Using a limited number of echocardiographic views, TEE appears ideally suited for the hemodynamic assessment of ventilated ICU patients. Although minimally invasive, TEE may result in rare oropharyngeal or esophageal complications. Recent miniaturization of TEE probe promises to increase its tolerance and further use this approach for the hemodynamic monitoring of the most unstable ventilated patients.

TABLE 5.3 Elements to consider before deciding the modality of critical care echocardiography for a diagnostic purpose

Transthoracic echocardiography (TTE)	Transesophageal echocardiography (TEE)
Systematically performed first due to noninvasiveness and ease of use	*Second intention*: nondiagnostic TTE *First intention*: higher diagnostic accuracy than TTE for the specific indications
TTE superior to TEE: superficial anatomical structures and orientation of jets • Suspected pericardial effusion (unloculated) and tamponade (tolerance), penetrating cardiac injury (hemopericardium) • Suspected thrombus of left ventricular apex • Identification of interventricular septal defect • Best Doppler beam alignment: Left ventricular outflow tract obstruction Aortic (prosthetic) valve pressure gradient Mitral (prosthetic) valve pressure gradient Evaluation of pulmonary artery pressure[a] • Guidance of invasive procedures (pericardiocentesis, external pacing)	*TEE superior to TTE*: deep-seated anatomical structures • Suspected pericardial loculated effusion or extrapericardial tamponade (compressive mediastinal hematoma[b]) after cardiac surgery or chest trauma • Mechanism and quantification of (prosthetic) mitral valve regurgitation • Suspected infective endocarditis • Suspected acute aortic disease (acute aortic syndrome, blunt aortic trauma) • Identification of embolus-in-transit or proximal pulmonary embolism[c] • Identification of cardiac or aortic source of systemic embolization • Identification of patent foramen ovale • Guidance of invasive procedure (stenting of the thoracic aorta, closure of patent foramen ovale, positioning of venous cannula of circulatory assistance or extracorporeal membrane oxygenation) • Complication of cardiac surgery, circulatory assistance or extracorporeal membrane oxygenation or of any endovascular procedure (e.g., stenting, patent foramen ovale closure)

[a]Based on tricuspid regurgitation
[b]The compressive hematoma is typically located posterior to the right atrium and less frequently near the left atrium
[c]In ventilated patients (tolerance)

Multiple Choice Questions

1. Critical care echocardiography:
    A. Is performed by a sonographer or a cardiologist and interpreted offline by a cardiologist
    B. Is performed and interpreted online by an intensivist at bedside
    C. Relies solely on transthoracic echocardiography
    D. Is used for immediate therapeutic management
    E. Is not adequately suited to monitor therapeutic interventions

    Answers: B, D

2. Transesophageal echocardiography:
    A. Is part of competence for performing advanced critical care echocardiography
    B. Is safe to perform in ventilated patients
    C. Is contraindicated in patients with esophageal diseases or unstable cervical spine injury
    D. Should be avoided in spontaneously breathing patients with respiratory compromise
    E. Has an overall superior diagnostic capacity than transthoracic echocardiography

    Answers: A, B, C, D, E

Suggested Readings

Begot E, Dalmay F, Etchecopar C, Clavel M, Pichon N, Francois B, Lang R, Vignon P. Hemodynamic assessment of ventilated ICU patients with cardiorespiratory failure using a miniaturized multiplane transesophageal echocardiography probe. Intensive Care Med. 2015;41(11):1886–94.

Cecconi M, De Backer D, Antonelli M, Beale R, Bakker J, Hofer C, Jaeschke R, Mebazaa A, Pinsky MR, Teboul JL, Vincent JL, Rhodes A. Consensus on circulatory shock and hemodynamic monitoring. Task force of the European Society of Intensive Care Medicine. Intensive Care Med. 2014;40(12):1795–815.

Chan KL, Cohen GI, Sochowski RA, Baird MG. Complications of transesophageal echocardiography in ambulatory adult patients: analysis of 1500 consecutive examinations. J Am Soc Echocardiogr. 1991;4(6):577–82.

Expert Round Table on Echocardiography in ICU. International consensus statement on training standards for advanced critical care echocardiography. Intensive Care Med. 2014;40(5):654–66.

Expert Round Table on Ultrasound in ICU. International expert statement on training standards for critical care ultrasonography. Intensive Care Med. 2011;37(7):1077–83.

Grumann A, Baretto L, Dugard A, Morera P, Cornu E, Amiel JB, Vignon P. Localized cardiac tamponade after open-heart surgery. Ann Thorac Cardiovasc Surg. 2012;18(6):524–9.

Hüttemann E, Schelenz C, Kara F, Chatzinikolaou K, Reinhart K. The use and safety of transoesophageal echocardiography in the general ICU – a minireview. Acta Anaesthesiol Scand. 2004;48(7):827–36.

Mayo P, Beaulieu Y, Doelken P, Feller-Kopman D, Harrod C, Kaplan A, Oropello J, Vieillard-Baron A, Axler O, Lichtenstein D, Maury E, Slama M, Vignon P. Chest. 2009;135(4):1050–60.

Vieillard-Baron A, Slama M, Mayo P, Charron C, Amiel JB, Esterez C, Leleu F, Repesse X, Vignon P. A pilot study on safety and clinical utility of a single-use 72-hour indwelling transesophageal echocardiography probe. Intensive Care Med. 2013;39(4):629–35.

Vieillard-Baron A, Naeije R, Haddad F, Bogaard HJ, Bull TM, Fletcher N, Lahm T, Magder S, Orde S, Schmidt G, Pinsky MR. Diagnostic workup, etiologies and management of acute right ventricle failure : A state-of-the-art paper. Intensive Care Med. 2018;44(6):774–90.

Vignon P, Repessé X, Bégot E, Léger J, Jacob C, Bouferrache K, Slama M, Prat G, Vieillard-Baron A. Comparison of Echocardiographic Indices Used to Predict Fluid Responsiveness in Ventilated Patients. Am J Respir Crit Care Med. 2017;195(8):1022–32.

Vignon P, Boncoeur MP, François B, Rambaud G, Maubon A, Gastinne H. Comparison of multiplane transesophageal echocardiography and contrast-enhanced helical CT in the diagnosis of blunt traumatic cardiovascular injuries. Anesthesiology. 2001;94(4):615–22.

Vignon P, Mentec H, Terré S, Gastinne H, Guéret P, Lemaire F. Diagnostic accuracy and therapeutic impact of transthoracic and transesophageal echocardiography in mechanically ventilated patients in the ICU. Chest. 1994;106(6):1829–34.

Vignon P, Begot E, Mari A, Silva S, Chimot L, Delour P, Vargas F, Filloux B, Vandroux D, Jabot J, François B, Pichon N, Clavel M, Levy B, Slama M, Riu-Poulenc B. Hemodynamic Assessment of Patients With Septic Shock Using Transpulmonary Thermodilution and Critical Care Echocardiography: A Comparative Study. Chest. 2018;153(1):55–64.

Vignon P, Merz TM, Vieillard-Baron A. Ten reasons for performing hemodynamic monitoring using transesophageal echocardiography. Intensive Care Med. 2017;43(7):1048–51.

Vignon P. What is new in critical care echocardiography? Crit Care. 2018;22(1):40.

Vignon P. Hemodynamic assessment of critically ill patients using echocardiography Doppler. Curr Opin Crit Care. 2005;11(3):227–34.

Chapter 6
Transthoracic Echocardiography: Technical Aspects

Michel Slama

Transthoracic echocardiography (TTE) should be done first before transesophageal echocardiography (TEE) at the bedside in ICU spontaneously breathing or mechanically ventilated patients using low-frequency or multifrequency probe. Parasternal, apical, and subcostal views should be performed. TTE could be performed from the right or left hand side of the bed (Table 6.1).

Loops: TTE with poor visualization and good visualization of vegetation…. Contrary for flow …

M. Slama (✉)
Medical ICU, CHU Sud, Amiens, France
e-mail: slama.michel@chu-amiens.fr

© Springer Nature Switzerland AG 2020
M. Slama (ed.), *Echocardiography in ICU*,
https://doi.org/10.1007/978-3-030-32219-9_6

83

TABLE 6.1 Advantages and disadvantages of transthoracic (TTE) and transesophageal echocardiography (TEE)

Advantages of TTE examination	Advantages of TEE examination
– Strictly noninvasive procedure – Visualization of the pericardium and guidance for pericardiocentesis – Visualization of left ventricular apex (suspicion of thrombus, apical myocardial infarction) – Visualization of interventricular septal defect – Visualization of inferior vena cava – Visualization of subhepatic veins – Good alignment with all intracardiac flows particularly to record tricuspid regurgitation, left ventricular obstructive flow, aortic regurgitant, and stenotic flows	– High imaging quality – Cardiac post op tamponade (suspected extracardiac tamponade, loculated compressive pericardial effusion) – Mechanisms and quantification of native or prosthetic mitral valve (quantification of mitral regurgitation, prosthesis evaluation) – Superior vena cava visualization – Assessment of interatrial defect of patent foramen ovale (intracardiac shunt) – Visualization of thoracic aorta (dissection, traumatic injury) – Visualization of left atrial appendage – Visualization of vegetation and cardiac abscess
Disadvantages of TTE examination	Disadvantages of TEE examination
– Nondiagnostic surface imaging (dressings, tubes, poor visualization of deep structure, obesity, lung hyperinflation, emphysema)	– Very rare but possible severe complications (esophageal perforation 1/2500)

Multiple Choice Questions

1. Transthoracic echocardiography should be a preferred route for the visualization of:

   A. Left atrial appendage
   B. Patent foramen ovale
   C. Left ventricular obstructive flow
   D. Left ventricular apical thrombus
   E. Mitral prosthetic valve
   Answers: C, D

2. Transesophageal echocardiography may provide a better visualization of:

   A. Left atrial appendage
   B. Left ventricular apex
   C. Tricuspid regurgitation flow maximal velocity
   D. Mitral prosthetic valve
   E. Ascending aorta
   Answers: A, D, E

Suggested Reading

Vignon P, Mayo P. Echocardiography in the critically ill: an overview. In: De Backer D, Cholley B, Slama M, Vieillard Baron A, Vignon P, editors. Hemodynamic monitoring using echocardiography in the critically ill. New York: Springer; 2011. p. 1–7.

Chapter 7
Transesophageal Echocardiography (TEE) in Mechanically Ventilated Patients: Practical Aspects

Michel Slama

TEE examination could be done either in a spontaneously breathing patient or in a patient under mechanical ventilation. Contraindications should be ruled out (Box 7.1). Information should be given to the patient, and consent should be obtained. In case of sedation or mechanical ventilation, the patient's next of kin should be informed (Boxes 7.2 and 7.3).

7.1 Description of the Probe

Classic multiplane TEE is usually used in ICU patients. Miniaturized probes or pediatric probe could be used in ICU patients as well. Nasal introduction could be done using these small probes permitting to perform in an easiest way TEE in nonintubated patients. Electronic rotation could be done using a knob on the probe from 0° to 180°. The tip of the

M. Slama (✉)
Medical ICU, CHU Sud, Amiens, France
e-mail: slama.michel@chu-amiens.fr

© Springer Nature Switzerland AG 2020
M. Slama (ed.), *Echocardiography in ICU*,
https://doi.org/10.1007/978-3-030-32219-9_7

Box 7.1 Transesophageal Echocardiography Contraindications

- *Absolute contraindications*
  - Any relevant esophageal or ENT disease (tumor, esophageal stenosis, diverticula, laceration, perforation...)
  - Mediastinal radiation therapy
  - Excessive risk of bleeding
  - Recent esophageal/upper GI or ENT surgery
  - Unstable neck fracture

- *Relative contraindications*
  - Nonempty stomach
  - Hemodynamically unstable spontaneously breathing patient
  - Acute respiratory failure in spontaneously breathing patient
  - Agitated and noncompliant patient
  - Esophageal noncontrolled hemorrhage or recent esophageal bleeding
  - History of nonexplored dysphasia

Box 7.2 Check List Before Transesophageal (TEE) Probe Insertion

- Inform the patient or the patient's next of kin concerning the procedure and the risks.
- Ask patient to fast for at least 4 h/empty stomach/ gastric liquid suction through gastric tube.
- Contraindications should be ruled out.
- The patient should have venous access.
- All needed materials should be prepared.
- TEE should be connected to the echo machine.
- ECG should be connected to the echo machine.
- Monitoring should be "on" (ECG, oxygen saturation, blood pressure).
- Withdraw any dental appliance.
- Nonintubated patients should be placed in left lateral decubitus position.

probe could be flexed laterally (smaller control wheel on the probe handle) and anteriorly and posteriorly (larger control wheel). Wheels could be locked or unlocked (Figs. 7.1 and 7.2).

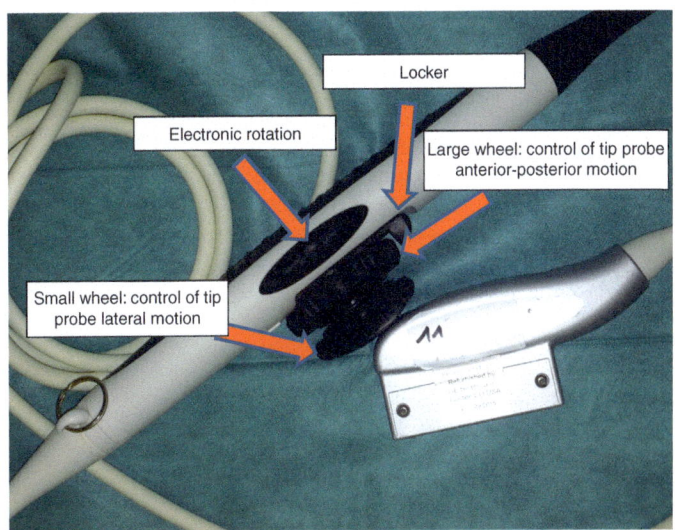

FIGURE 7.1 TEE probe

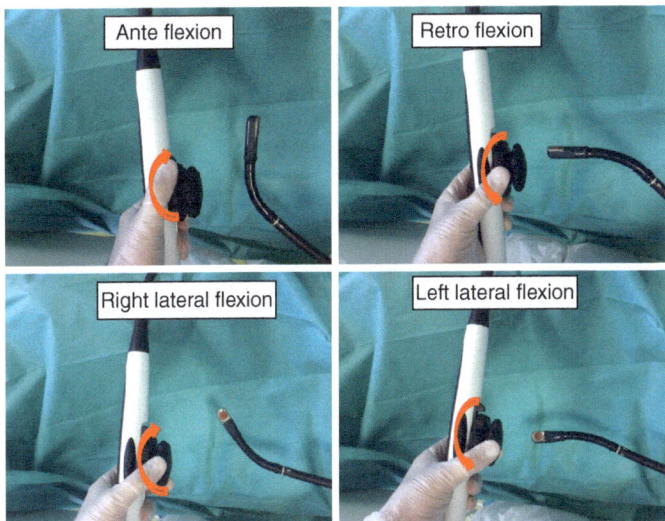

FIGURE 7.2 Motion control of the probe tip

Box 7.3 Practical Aspects of TEE Examination

- The echocardiographer stands facing the patient on the left-hand side (or right) of the bed.
- The echocardiographic machine with ECG (and respiratory) signal displayed on the echo screen should be placed in front of the echocardiographer.
- The probe should be in an unlocked position.
- Local anesthetic agent (Lidocaïn®)/sedation, and/or neuromuscular blocking agents should be prepared.
- Allergy to these drugs should be ruled out.
- At least a nurse should assist during the procedure.

Box 7.4 Materials for Transesophageal (TEE) Echocardiography (Fig. 7.3)

- TEE probe
- Bite block
- Topical anesthetic agent (Xylocaïn)/sedation, and/or neuromuscular blocking agents
- Syringe, needle, and taps
- Gloves
- Saline (for contrast examination)
- Laryngoscope
- Protective glasses
- All materials for resuscitation

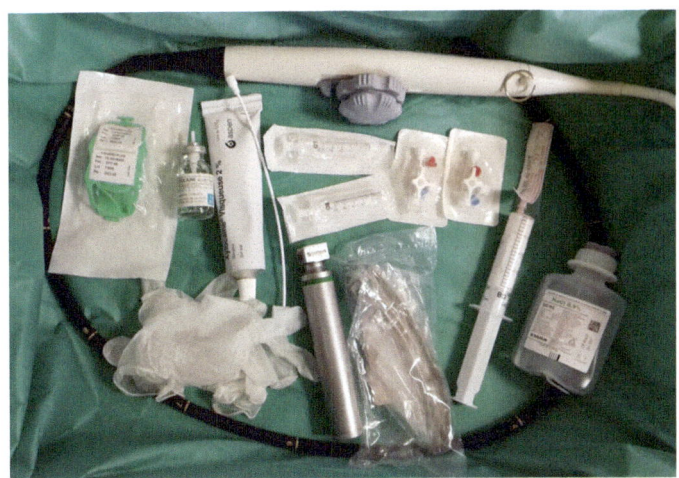

FIGURE 7.3 Materials that should be prepared for transesophageal echocardiography (TEE)

7.2   TEE Examination

TEE in spontaneously breathing patients should be done in a lateral position (Fig. 7.4). Topical anesthesia should be done, and sometimes light sedation could help. TEE probe is introduced via a bite block to the back of the pharynx (Box 7.4, Fig. 7.3). Then the patient should swallow; meanwhile, the operator should introduce gently the probe into the esophagus.

TEE in mechanically ventilated patients should be done under sedation and sometimes after injection of neuromuscular blocking agents. The patient should be in supine position with the head at 30°. The probe is usually introduced blindly or under direct laryngoscopy (Box 7.5).

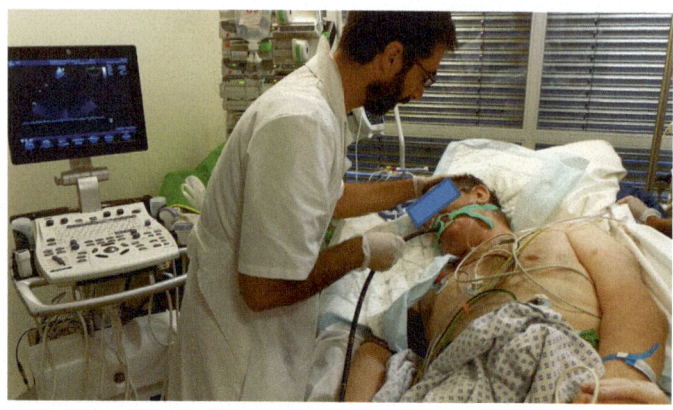

FIGURE 7.4 Blind introduction of the TEE probe in spontaneously breathing patients

---

Box 7.5 Tricks to Make Easier Transesophageal (TEE) Probe Introduction

What to do in case of unsuccessful blind introduction of the TEE probe in mechanically ventilated patients.

- Check sedation and inject neuromuscular blocking agents (if no contraindication).
- Insert one or two fingers into the mouth and guide the probe toward the midline and depress the tongue if it is blocking passage.
- Flex the neck anteriorly.
- Lift the mandible anteriorly.
- Introduce the TEE probe under direct visualization using laryngoscopy.

7.3   Complications of TEE Examination

Rate of complication is very low (0.18–2.8%) except for small buccal hemorrhage and gastric tube dislodgement, especially during probe withdrawal (Table 7.1). Mortality was reported in cardiologic field (<0.01–0.02%) but neither in ICU nor

TABLE 7.1 Transesophageal procedure complications, risk factors, and prevention

Complications	Clinical situations	Precautions
Esophageal trauma or perforation (exceptional: 1/2500 TEE examination)	ENT/esophageal disease	ENT examination/ esophagogastroscopie in case of doubt
	Small patient	Use pediatric or a small TEE probe
Aortic rupture (exceptional)	Aortic dissection	Avoid blood pressure rise and/or sedation and mechanical ventilation
Peripheral embolism or stroke (exceptional)	Large thrombus in a large left atrium or in aortic aneurysm	Avoid tip TEE probe lateral and anterior-posterior motion
Buccal hemorrhage/ dental trauma (frequent)	Difficult TEE introduction	Use laryngoscopy for the introduction of the probe
Esophageal hemorrhage (rare)	Hemostasis disorder	Prevention
Cardiac arrhythmia (rare)	Hemodynamically instable patient/ ischemic cardiomyopathy	Correction of risk factors (ischemia, fever, hypokalemia, hypoxemia)
Dislodgement of endotracheal tube or gastric tube (frequent)	Hard TEE probe motion/ patient agitation, especially on probe withdrawal	Have an gentle motion of the TEE probe during the examination/ patient sedation
Aspiration (rare)	Unconscious nonintubated patients/swallowing disorder	Tracheal intubation to prevent aspiration

during intraoperative TEE. Bronchospasme and laryngo-spasme were reported in 0.02% and 0.14% in cardiologic field but never in ICU patients.

Multiple Choice Questions

1. Among these situations, which are absolute contraindications of a TEE examination?

    A. Cerebral ischemic stroke
    B. Septic shock in mechanically ventilated patients
    C. Mediastinal radiation therapy
    D. Esophageal tumor
    E. Unstable cervical trauma
    Answers: C, D, E

2. About TEE complications, give the right answers:

    A. TEE severe complications are frequent >10%
    B. TEE severe complications are rare in ICU and during perioperative period <3%
    C. Esophageal perforation may occur during TEE examination but is very rare
    D. Dislodgement of gastric tube is frequent
    E. Severe endocarditis may occur due to TEE examination
    Answers: B, C, D

3. In case of failure of blind TEE probe insertion, we may:

    A. Push strongly the probe blindly
    B. Do a neck flexion
    C. Lift the mandible posteriorly
    D. Put two fingers in the mouth to guide the probe
    E. Inject paralytic agent
    Answers: B, D, E

Suggested Readings

Hahn R. Guidelines for performing a comprehensive transesophageal echocardiographic examination: recommendations from the American Society of Echocardiography and the Society of Cardiovascular Anesthesiologists. J Am Soc Echocardiogr. 2013;26:921–64.

Vignon P, Mayo P. Echocardiography in the critically ill: an overview. In: De Backer D, Cholley B, Slama M, Vieillard Baron A, Vignon P, editors. Hemodynamic monitoring using echocardiography in the critically ill. New York: Springer; 2011. p. 1–7.

Part III
Heart Lung Interactions

Chapter 8
Heart–Lung Interactions

Antoine Vieillard-Baron

Heart–lung interaction evaluation largely participates in the hemodynamic evaluation of critically ill patients, especially when patients are mechanically ventilated. In patients in shock with pulse pressure variations (PPV), transesophageal echocardiography allows to determine the mechanism of such variations, guiding the treatment (Figs. 8.1 and 8.2).

The following proposed *algorithm* was not strictly validated per se but is based on physiology, clinical studies in the field, and the experience of the author.

The previous algorithm requires only four simple following echocardiographic views (Figs. 8.3, 8.4, 8.5, and 8.6) with their related parameters to be applied when PPV is used as a "warning" signal.

A. Vieillard-Baron (✉)
Surgical and Medical ICU, University Hospital Ambroise Paré,
APHP, Boulogne-Billancourt, France
e-mail: antoine.vieillard-baron@aphp.fr

© Springer Nature Switzerland AG 2020   99
M. Slama (ed.), *Echocardiography in ICU*,
https://doi.org/10.1007/978-3-030-32219-9_8

a

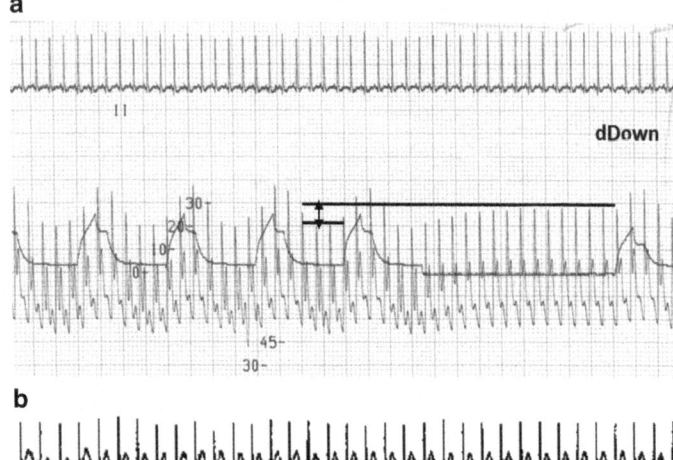

b

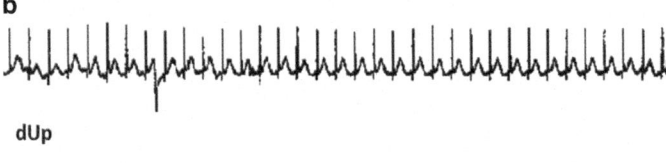

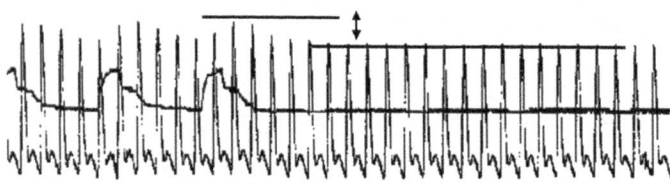

FIGURE 8.1 Pulse pressure variations (PPV). (**a**) dDown effect; (**b**) dUp effect

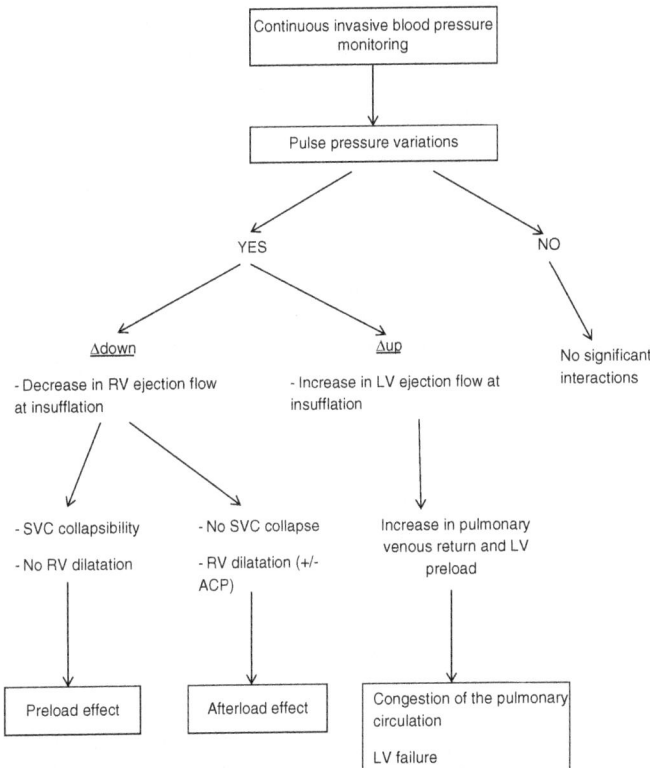

FIGURE 8.2 Algorithm management starting from pulse pressure variations (PPV). *ACP* acute cor pulmonale, *RV* right ventricle, *LV* left ventricle

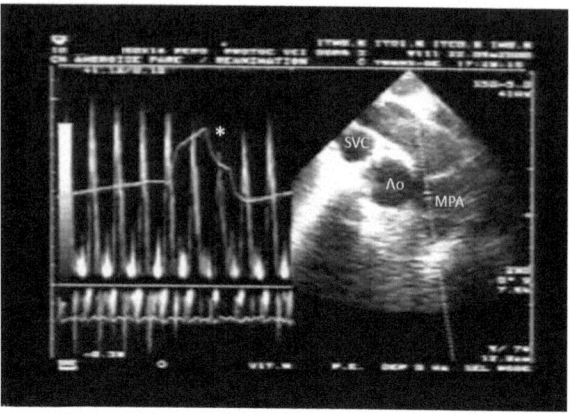

FIGURE 8.3 Transverse (0°) upper esophageal view, 25–30 cm under the dental arch. It allows putting the pulsed wave Doppler (PWD) sample into the main pulmonary artery to record any respiratory changes of the right ventricular (RV) ejection flow during the respiratory cycle. In case of dDown, a significant decrease during tidal ventilation is observed (*). *SVC*: superiorvena cava; *Ao*: ascending aorta; *MPA*: main pulmonary artery

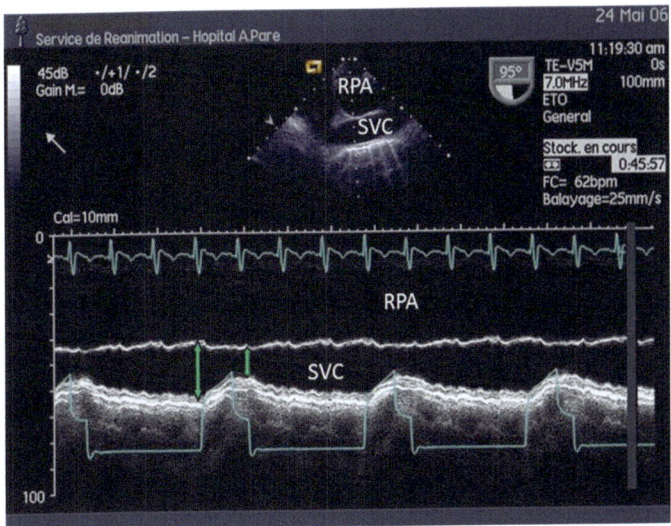

FIGURE 8.4 Longitudinal view of the superior vena cava (SVC). From view number 1, the SVC is placed in the center of the screen of the echo machine, and the ultrasound beam is rotated at 90°. In case of partial or complete SVC collapse during tidal ventilation visualized using the time motion study, it is very likely that hemodynamics will be improved by fluid expansion. This reflects the "preload effect" of mechanical ventilation. *RPA*: right pulmonary artery

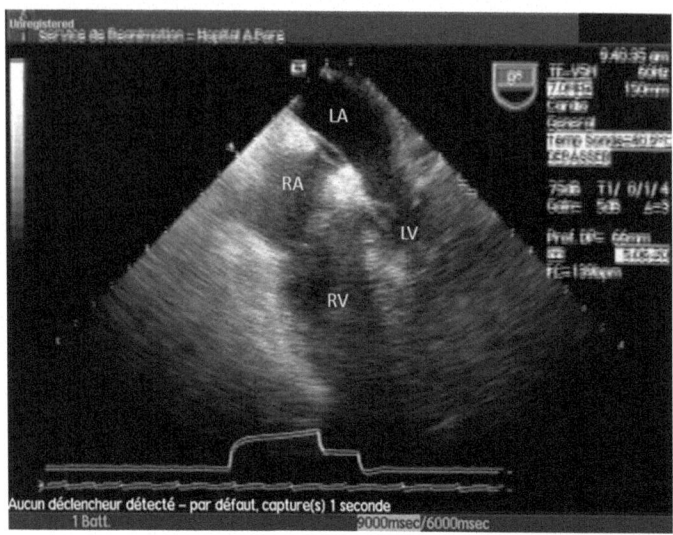

FIGURE 8.5 Transverse mid-esophageal view, 30–35 cm under the dental arch. It allows physicians to evaluate the size of the right ventricle. In case of dDown, when the SVC does not vary with the respiration and the right ventricle is dilated (visually or when the ratio between the end-diastolic areas of the right and the left ventricle is higher than 0.6), this reflects an "afterload effect" of mechanical ventilation. In this case, this is very unlikely that hemodynamics improve with more fluids, and the right ventricle must be supported

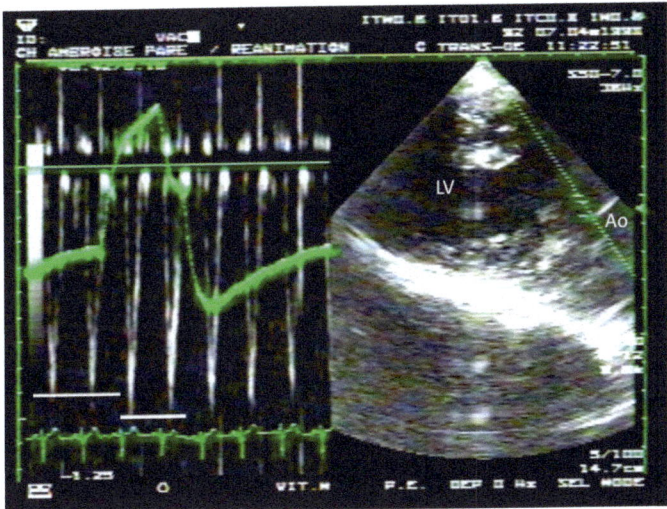

FIGURE 8.6 Left ventricular outflow track from the transverse transgastric view, 40–45 cm under the dental arch. From this view, the ultrasound beam is rotated until 100–110° and the PWD sample is placed into the LV outflow track. In case of isolated dUp, an increase in the LV flow is observed during tidal ventilation without any respiratory variation of the SVC or without RV dilatation. This usually reflects a high amount of blood into the pulmonary circulation leading to an increased pulmonary venous return and LV preload by tidal ventilation; the respiratory status may be improved by fluid removal

Multiple Choice Questions

1. In case of dDown, TEE may visualize:

   A. A major RV dilatation.
   B. The absence of respiratory variation of the RV ejection flow.
   C. A complete collapse of the SVC during expiration.
   D. A complete collapse of the SVC during insufflation.
   E. A massive mitral regurgitation.

   Answers: A, D

2. To analyze the SVC:

    A. A TEE is required.
    B. A TTE is required.
    C. The subcostal view is the optimal one.
    D. An upper esophageal view has to be obtained.
    E. The pulsed wave Doppler mode is mandatory.
    Answers: A, D

3. A TEE performed in a patient with a dUP may visualize:

    A. An inspiratory collapse of the SVC.
    B. An acute cor pulmonale.
    C. An increase in pulmonary venous return during insufflation.
    D. An increase in LV ejection flow during expiration.
    E. An increase in LV ejection flow during insufflation.
    Answers: C, E

Suggested Readings

Jardin F, Farcot JC, Gueret P, et al. Cyrclic changes in arterial pulse during respiratory support. Circulation. 1983;68:266–74.

Massumi R, Mason D, Zakauddin V, et al. Reversed pulsus paradoxus. N Engl J Med. 1976;289:1272–5.

Michard F, Boussat S, Chemla D, et al. Relation between respiratory changes in arterial pulse pressure and fluid responsiveness in septic patients. Am J Respir Crit Care Med. 2000;162:134–8.

Perel A, Pizov R, Cotev S. Systolic blood pressure variations is a sensitive indicator of hypovolemia in ventilated dog subject to graded hemorrhage. Anesthesiology. 1987;67:498–502.

Versprille A. The pulmonary circulation during mechanical ventilation. Acta Anaesthesiol Scand. 1990;34:51–62.

Vieillard-Baron A, Chergui K, Augarde R, et al. Cyclic changes in arterial pulse during respiratory support revisited by Doppler echocardiography. Am J Respir Crit Care Med. 2003;168:671–6.

Part IV
Hemodynamic Evaluation

Chapter 9
Fluid Requirement and Fluid Responsiveness

Michel Slama

Fluid therapy is the cornerstone of hemodynamic resuscitation. It is demonstrated that positive fluid balance could be associated with a poor prognosis of ARDS and septic shock patients. Also, hypovolemia is associated with tissue hypoperfusion and should be corrected by volume expansion. Then volume expansion should be considered as a drug. A restrictive administration should be preferred. Volume expansion will be considered in case of a clinical situation associated with tissue hypoperfusion. Because clinical signs are neither sensitive nor specific to predict fluid responsiveness, echocardiographic parameters were developed to better predict fluid needs.

───────
Electronic Supplementary Material The online version of this chapter (https://doi.org/10.1007/978-3-030-32219-9_9) contains supplementary material, which is available to authorized users.

───────
M. Slama (✉)
Medical ICU, CHU Sud, Amiens, France
e-mail: slama.michel@chu-amiens.fr

9.1   Static Indices Based on Preload Assessment

Preload is defined as the size of the ventricle at end diastole. Relationship between preload and stroke volume is called Franck-Starling relationship. Echocardiographic static indices of fluid (Box 9.1) needs as based on preload assessment. This concept states that if the preload is low, then increasing the preload with volume expansion would increase stroke volume and cardiac output (responder patient). In contrast, in case of high preload, any change of this preload will not be associated with stroke volume and or cardiac output change (nonresponder patient).

Box 9.1 Fluid Responsiveness: Static Parameters

Static parameters of positive fluid responsiveness

Left ventricle (LV): small LV using visual evaluation, small LV diameter (parasternal long-axis view M-mode or 2D measurement): woman <3.9 cm, 2.4 cm/m^2; men <4.2 cm, 2.2 cm/m^2, small LV area (parasternal short-axis view): <5.5 cm/m^2, small LV volume (Simpson method from apical view): women <56 ml, <35 ml/m^2; men <67 ml, <35 ml/m^2

Left ventricular hyperkinesia: visual hyperkinesia, kissing wall, measured hyperkinesia: ejection fraction (apical view) >70%, shortening fraction >45% woman, >43% man

Pseudo LV hypertrophy: small left ventricle and increased wall thickness with normal-calculated LV mass

LV obstruction with systolic anterior motion, premature cloture of the aortic valve, and LV obstructive flow recorded using continuous wave Doppler (from the apical five-chamber view; this flow should be researched with attention because it is difficult to record). High positive predictive value (Fig. 9.1) (Case 3 loop 1 kissing wall A4C with obstruction)

Small right ventricle (almost virtual) (Case 1 loops 1, 2, 3. LV hyperkinesia with kissing walls respectively from parasternal long axis, short-axis view, and apical 4-chamber view) (Case 4 loop 1 hypovolemia kissing wall parasternal short-axis view), left atrium, and right atrium

Small inferior vena cava (IVC). Expiratory diameter ≤10 mm (≥27 mmHg predict nonresponders, between 10 and 27 grey zone). High predictive value (Case 2 Loop 1 hypovolemia IVC inspiration)

9.2   Dynamic Parameters to Predict Fluid Responsiveness Based on Heart–Lung Interactions

Dynamic parameters use a maneuver that test Franck Starling relationship. Heart–lung interactions are used to assess fluid responsiveness when we record IVC, SVC, and aortic blood flow and when we perform an inspiratory/expiratory maneuver. Other parameters are not based on heart–lung interaction as passive leg raising maneuver and mini fluid challenge increase the cardiac preload to test the heart response by assessing left ventricular ejection (aortic VTI, stroke volume, cardiac output) (Tables 9.1 and 9.2).

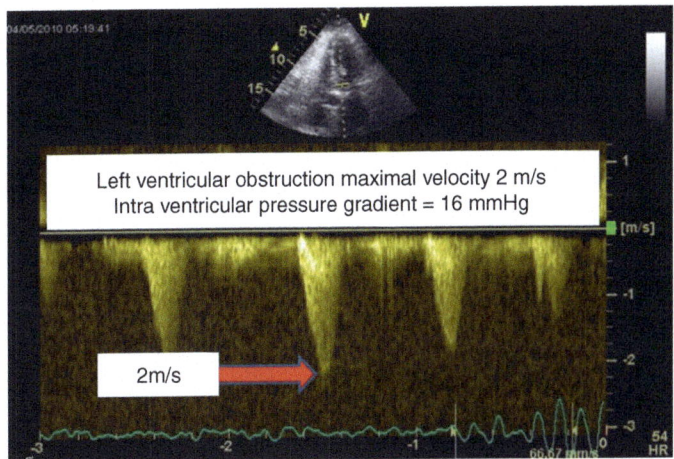

FIGURE 9.1 Left ventricular obstruction

TABLE 9.1 Dynamic parameters to predict fluid responsiveness based on heart–lung interactions

Parameters	Technical aspect/ recording	TTE/ TEE	MV/SB	Equation	Fluid responder, %	Limits
IVC distensibility Index (Fig. 9.2)	From subcostal view 2–3 cm away from the right atrium avoiding subhepatic vein M-mode	TTE	MV	(IVCexp-IVCinsp)/ IVC exp	>13	High PEEP low TV, inspiratory effort, lung hyperinflation, increased abdominal pressure, misalignment due to marked IVC respiratory translation motion, IVC thrombus compression…)
IVC collapsibility index (Fig. 9.3)	From subcostal view 2–3 cm away from the right atrium avoiding subhepatic vein M-mode	TTE	SB	(IVCexp-IVCinsp)/ IVCexp	>45	High PEEP low TV, inspiratory effort, lung hyperinflation, increased abdominal pressure, misalignment due to marked IVC respiratory translation motion, IVC thrombus compression…)
			SB. Deep calibrated inspiration −5 cm to −10 H_2O during 5 s	(IVCexp-IVCinsp)/ IVCexp	>50	

Method	Technique	TTE or TEE	MV	Formula	Threshold	Limitations
Aortic blood flow respiratory changes (Fig. 9.4)	Pulsed Doppler sample volume behind aortic valves	TTE or TEE	MV	$(V_{max} - V_{min})/V_{mean}$ $aoVTI_{max}-aoVTI_{min})/aoVTI_{mean}$	>13 >20	Arrhythmia, RV dilation or dysfunction, low tidal volume, high intraabdominal pressure
SVC collapsibility (Fig. 9.5)	90° using M-mode	TTE	MV	$(SVC_{max}-SVC_{min})/SVC_{max}$	>21	Low tidal volume
End-expiratory maneuver	Aortic blood flow recording	TTE	MV	aoVTI before/aoVTI during end expiration	>10	None
End-expiratory and inspiratory maneuver	Aortic blood flow recording	TTE	MV	aoVTI percentage changes	>13	None

MV mechanical ventilation, *SB* spontaneously breathing, *VTI* velocity time integral, *IVC* inferior vena cava, *SVC* superior vena cava, *V* velocity

TABLE 9.2 Dynamic parameters to predict fluid responsiveness not based on heart–lung interactions

Parameters	Technical aspect/ recording	TTE/ TEE	MV/ SB	Equation	Fluid responder, %	Limits
Passive leg raising (Fig. 9.6)	Moving the bed from semi-recumbent position to supine position with leg raising Either VTI, SV, CO, or CI recorded 1 mn after mobilization	TTE/ TEE	MV/ SB	(aoVTI before – aoVTI during)/aoVTI before	>10	Intraabdominal hypertension, compressive socks, caution in patients with severe intracranial hypertension
Mini-fluid challenge	100 ml hydroxyethyl starch infusion over 1 min, aoVTI	TTE	MV/ SB	(aoVTI before – aoVTI during)/aoVTI before	≥10	None
	50 ml crystalloid solution				≥10	None
Fluid challenge	Volume expansion 250–500 ml over 10–15 mn	TTE/ TEE	MV/ SB	(aoVTI before – aoVTI during)/aoVTI before	>15	None

Right ventricular dilation and dysfunction is usually a contraindication to volume expansion (Box 9.2).

Box 9.2 When Stopping Volume Expansion?

When stopping volume expansion?

Clinical goal reached

Disappearance of tissue hypoperfusion clinical and/or biological signs

Absence of fluid-responsiveness echocardiographic signs

No change of either stroke volume or cardiac output after fluid challenge

Clinical signs of bad tolerance

Echocardiographic evidence of either high left filling pressure or right ventricular dysfunction

Apparition of B lines on lung ultrasound

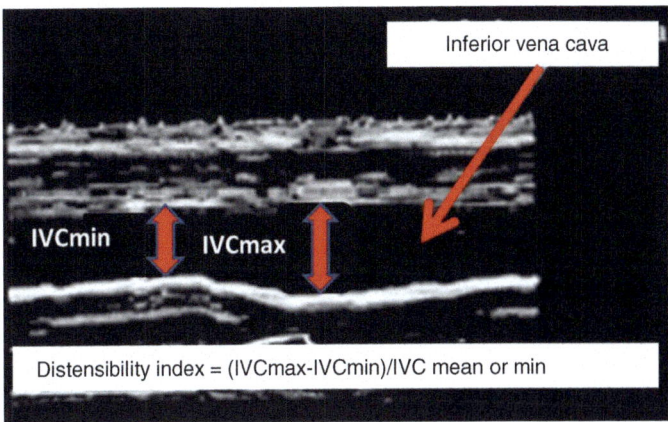

FIGURE 9.2 Inferior vena cava distensibility index in patients under mechanical ventilation

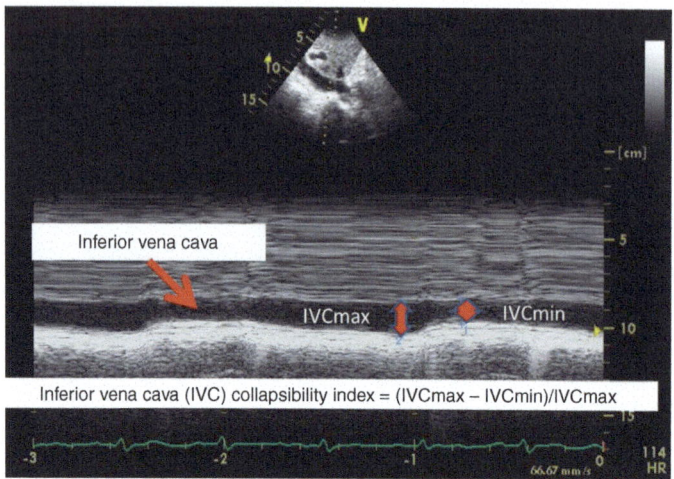

FIGURE 9.3 Inferior vena cava collapsibility index in spontaneously breathing patients

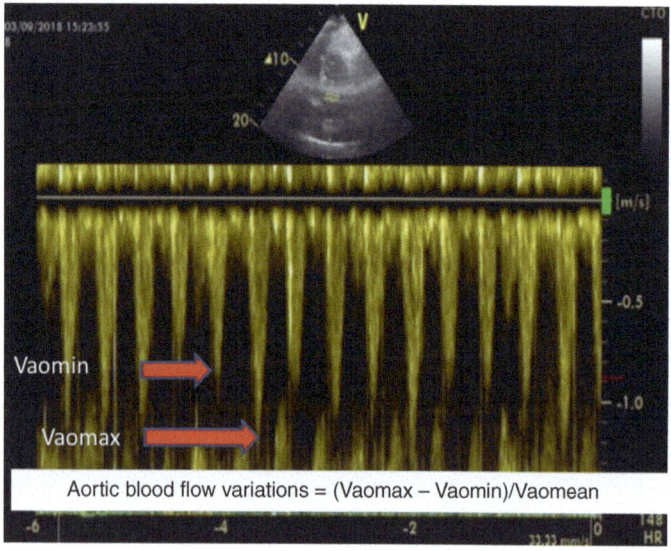

FIGURE 9.4 Measurement of aortic blood flow respiratory variations. Maximal (Vaomax) and minimal (Vaomin) velocities are measured, and mean (Vaomean) is calculated from maximal and minimal velocities ((Vaomax + Vaomin)/2)

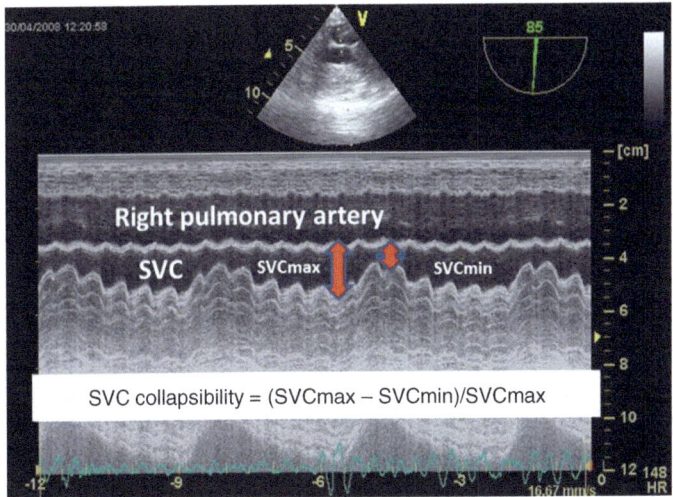

FIGURE 9.5 Superior vena cava (SVC) collapsibility index assessment

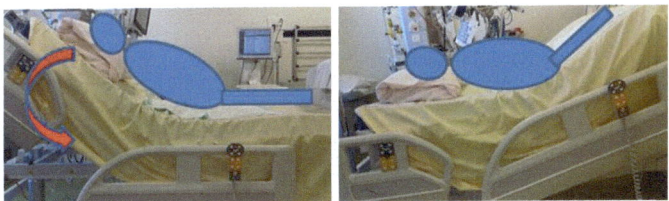

FIGURE 9.6 Passive leg raising maneuver

Multiple Choice Questions

1. The following observation in septic shock patients predict fluid responsiveness:

   A. Left ventricular obstruction.
   B. Large left ventricle.
   C. Very small inferior vena cava.
   D. Left ventricular hypokinesia.
   E. Left ventricular kissing wall.
   Answers: A, C, E

2. In case of atrial fibrillation, we should use the following parameters to assess fluid responsiveness:

   A. Aortic blood flow velocity respiratory variations.
   B. Aortic blood flow VTI respiratory variations.
   C. Superior vena cava respiratory variations.
   D. Mitral flow velocity respiratory variations.
   E. Tricuspid regurgitation velocity.
   Answer: C

3. Passive leg raising maneuver:

   A. Is a strong predictive index of fluid responsiveness.
   B. Cannot be performed in spontaneously breathing patients.
   C. Cannot be used in patients under mechanical ventilation.
   D. Has a limited value in patients with high intraabdominal pressure.
   E. Cannot be used in atrial fibrillation.
   Answers: A, D

4. When a patient is under mechanical ventilation, we may use to assess fluid responsiveness:

   A. Superior vena cava distensibility index.
   B. Inferior vena cava distensibility index.
   C. Inferior vena cava collapsibility index.
   D. Superior vena cava collapsibility index.
   E. Passive leg raising.
   Answers: B, D, E

Loops/Cases

Case 1:

- Loop 1: parasternal long axis view of a patient with septic shock and severe hypovolemia. Left ventricle is small and hyperkinetic with almost a kissing wall.
- Loop 2: parasternal short axis view of a patient with septic shock and severe hypovolemia. Left ventricle is small and hyperkinetic with almost a kissing wall.

- Loop 3: apical four chamber view of a patient with septic shock and severe hypovolemia. Left ventricle is small and hyperkinetic with almost a kissing wall.

Case 2:

- Loop 1: inferior vena cava subcostal view of patient with shock under mechanical ventilation. Inferior vena cava is almost collapsed and the size of the IVC decreases during inspiration.

Case 3:

- Loop 1: apical four chamber view of patient with septic shock. We may observe a left ventricular hypertrophy with left ventricular obstruction and systolic anterior motion of the mitral valve.

Case 4:

- Loop 1: parasternal short axis view. Patient with severe hypovolemia kissing wall.

Suggested Readings

Boissier F, Razazi K, Seemann A, Bedet A, Thille AW, de Prost N, Lim P, Brun-Buisson C, Mekontso Dessap A. Left ventricular systolic dysfunction during septic shock: the role of loading conditions. Intensive Care Med. 2017;43(5):633–42.

Lang RM, Badano LP, Mor-Avi V, Afilalo J, Armstrong A, Ernande L, Flachskampf FA, Foster E, Goldstein SA, Kuznetsova T, Lancellotti P, Muraru D, Picard MH, Rietzschel ER, Rudski L, Spencer KT, Tsang W, Voigt JU. Recommendations for cardiac chamber quantification by echocardiography in adults: an update from the American Society of Echocardiography and the European Association of Cardiovascular Imaging. J Am Soc Echocardiogr. 2015;28(1):1–39.

Muller L, Toumi M, Bousquet PJ, Riu-Poulenc B, Louart G, Candela D, Zoric L, Suehs C, de La Coussaye JE, Molinari N, Lefrant JY, AzuRéa Group. An increase in aortic blood flow after an infusion of 100 ml colloid over 1 minute can predict fluid responsiveness: the mini-fluid challenge study. Anesthesiology. 2011;115(3):541–7.

Slama M, Maizel J. Assessment of fluid requirements: fluid responsiveness. In: De Backer D, Cholley B, Slama M, Vieilard-Baron A, Vignon PH, editors. Hemodynamic monitoring using echocardiography in the critically ill. Berlin: Springer; 2011. p. 31–69.

Slama M, Tribouilloy C, Maizel J. Left ventricular outflow tract obstruction in ICU patients. Curr Opin Crit Care. 2016;22(3):260–6.

Wu Y, Zhou S, Zhou Z, Liu B. A 10-second fluid challenge guided by transthoracic echocardiography can predict fluid responsiveness. Crit Care. 2014;18(3):R108.

Chapter 10
LV Global and Segmental Systolic Function Including Cardiac Output

Daniel De Backer

Evaluation of left ventricular function and cardiac output are key hemodynamic measurements.

10.1 Preamble

Even though physiologically linked, cardiac output and LV function can be dissociated: cardiac output can be preserved in case of impaired cardiac function, thanks to a decrease in afterload and an increase in preload. On the other hand, cardiac output can be decreased in case of increased afterload or decreased preload, even though contractility is preserved. Accordingly, when measuring cardiac output, it is important to also evaluate cardiac preload, afterload, and contractility. When measuring contractility, it is also important to measure stroke volume and cardiac output in order to evaluate the consequences of impaired contractility.

D. De Backer (✉)
Department of Intensive Care, CHIREC Hospitals, Université Libre de Bruxelles, Brussels, Belgium
e-mail: ddebacke@ulb.ac.be

© Springer Nature Switzerland AG 2020
M. Slama (ed.), *Echocardiography in ICU*,
https://doi.org/10.1007/978-3-030-32219-9_10

Many indices of cardiac contractility are preload and afterload sensitive. It is thus interesting to also evaluate cardiac preload and afterload, together with contractility and cardiac output.

10.2   Measurement of Cardiac Output

Cardiac output is computed as stroke volume times heart rate. Echocardiographic techniques thus attempt to measure stroke volume.

The most commonly used and also the most accurate method is based on the measurement of flow velocity at the level of the left ventricular outflow tract (LVOT). Stroke volume is computed as the product of the diameter of the LVOT (cm^2), and stroke distance is computed as the velocity time integral of aortic flow (VTIao, expressed in cm) (Fig. 10.1a, b). Great care should be taken to measure LVOT diameter, as a small error is put to the square, as well as to have excellent alignment of ultrasound beam and aortic flow. Ideally, 3–5 measurements should be averaged. Aortic stenosis and dynamic obstruction of LVOT affect reliability of measurements. Similarly, significant aortic regurgitation affects stroke volume measurements as some part of the ejected volume would regurgitate into the left ventricle.

Stroke volume can also be measured by estimation of end-systolic and end-diastolic volumes (usually by Simpson's method; see below). This technique is less reliable so that it is used only when the other methods cannot be used. It is also affected by aortic and mitral regurgitations but not by aortic stenosis.

Atrial fibrillation makes measurements of cardiac output more complicated due to the beat-by-beat variability of stroke volume. In atrial fibrillation, 10–13 consecutive beats should be averaged.

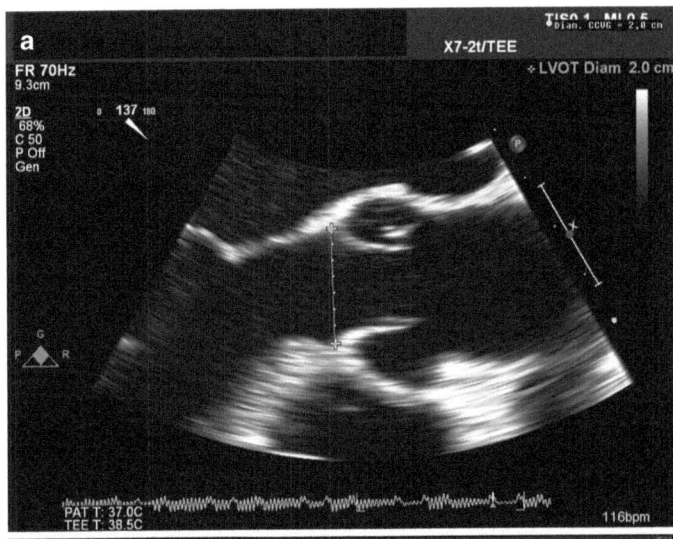

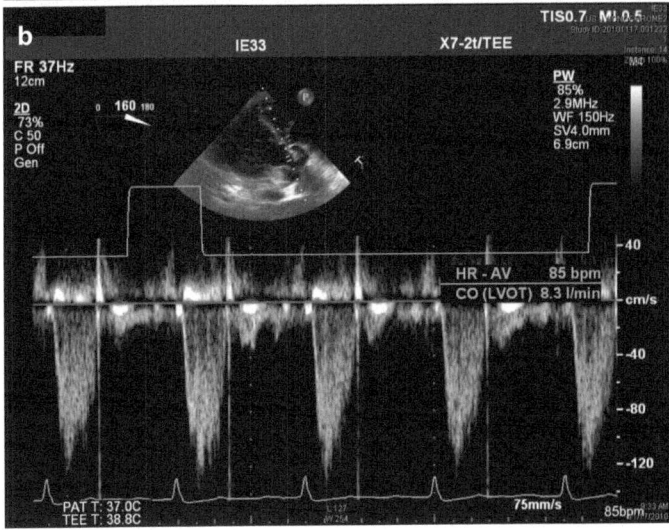

FIGURE 10.1 Measurement of cardiac output. Panel (**a**): Measurement of left ventricular outflow tract diameter. Panel (**b**): Measurement or aortic flow velocity time integral (VTIao). Cardiac output is computed as $3.1416 \times (LVOT\ diam/2)^2 \times VTIao \times heart\ rate$

10.3   Evaluation of LV Contractility

Several techniques can be used to evaluate LV contractility (Table 10.1).

TABLE 10.1 Techniques used to evaluate LV contractility

Measurement	TTE views	TEE views	Interpretation
Ejection fraction			
– Fractional area changes (measured or eyeball)	Parasternal short axis	Transgastric short axis	Nl > 60 Mild 40–50% Moderate 30–40% Severe <30%
– Simpson's	Apical 4- + 2-chamber views	Longitudinal ME	Nl >60 Mild 40–50% Moderate 30–40% Severe <30%
Displacement of mitral annulus			
– MAPSE	Apical 4-chamber (TM mode)	Longitudinal ME (TM mode)	Nl > 11 mm Severe <6 mm
– S wave	Apical 4 chambers (TDI)	Longitudinal ME (TDI)	Nl > 10 (septal) 8 (median) 9 (mean) cm/s
Mitral regurgitant flow dP/dT	Apical 4 chambers (CW)	Longitudinal ME (CW)	Nl 1200 mmHg/s
Speckle tracking (global longitudinal strain)	Apical 2, 3, and 4 chambers	Not available	Nl > −20 Severe < −10

ME mid-esophageal, *UE* upper esophageal, *Nl* normal, *TM* time motion, *TDI* tissue Doppler imaging, *CW* continuous wave Doppler, *MAPSE* mitral annulus plane systolic excursion

10.3.1   Ejection Fraction

Ejection fraction is the ratio between stroke volume and end-diastolic volume and can be estimated using several methods. One of the most important limitations of most measurements is that echography evaluates volumes from bi-dimensional views. Shortening fraction is computed as end-diastolic minus end-systolic diameters divided by end-diastolic diameter, with all diameters measured in time-motion mode. To be reliable, shortening fraction requires that contractility is homogeneous.

Ejection fraction can be estimated from fractional area changes at the level of papillary muscles. Fractional area change is either measured delineating the endocardial borders at end systole and end diastole or visually estimated (eyeball evaluation). Many studies have shown that eyeball estimation is reliable. Importantly, it should be measured at the level of the papillary muscle where it represents the average shortening of the ventricle (LV shortening increases from base to apex). Circumferential ejection fraction is representative of global ejection fraction as 80–90% of ventricular stroke volume is related to circumferential shortening. It is nevertheless less reliable when apical hypocontracility occurs, such as in Tako-Tsubo.

The Simpson method is methodologically the most reliable as it will approximate ejection fraction by volumetric estimations done on two perpendicular planes (apical 4- and 2-chamber views). This method use the principle of multiple disk summation (Fig. 10.2) and takes into account regional motion abnormalities. The major limitation of this technique is that small errors in endocardial delineation can induce significant errors in measurements.

Recent advances in technology allow the automated detection of endocardial borders and the computation of ejection fraction (Fig. 10.3).

10.3.2   MAPSE and Tissue Doppler

These two indices evaluate the systolic excursion of the mitral annulus, either by M-Mode (MAPSE for mitral annulus plane

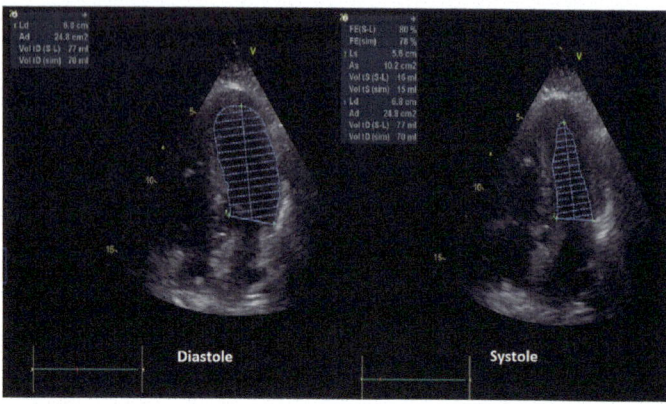

FIGURE 10.2 Simpson's method for measuring ejection fraction

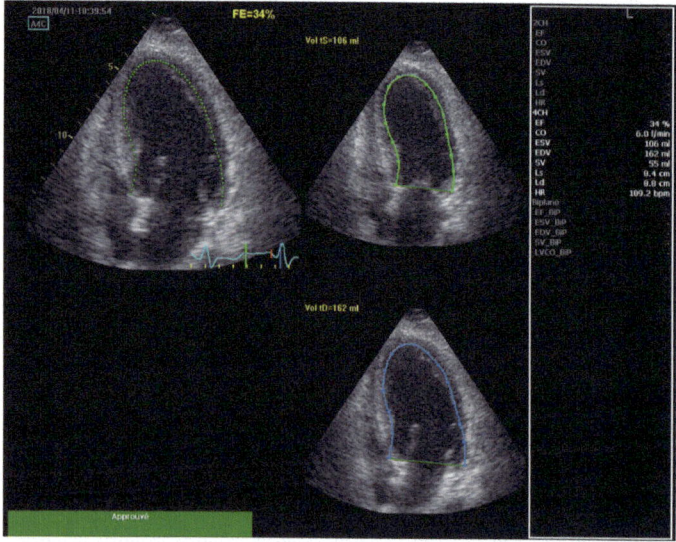

FIGURE 10.3 Ejection fraction obtained by automated border detection. This method is derived from Simpson's method, with automated border detection

systolic excursion) or by tissue Doppler (S wave) (Fig. 10.4). The main assumption is that longitudinal contraction reflects global systolic contraction. While this assumption is valid in

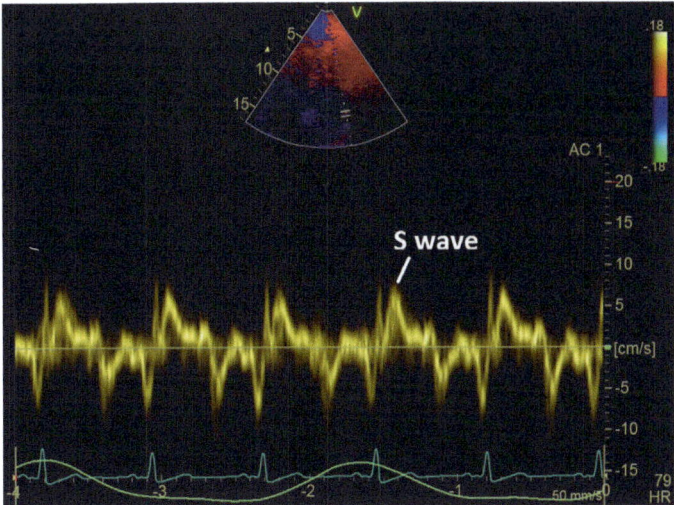

FIGURE 10.4 S wave of lateral mitral annulus on tissue Doppler. Obtained on apical 4-chamber view

many instances, these indices may not be valid in conditions with apical hypokinesia, such as Tako-Tsubo or ventricular aneurism, or with asynchrony.

The measurements are obtained at the level of the lateral and median part of mitral annulus in apical four chambers.

10.3.3   dP/dT$_{max}$

The LV dP/dT$_{max}$ is obtained from mitral regurgitant jet, and it represents the peak of the first derivative of systolic pressure rise of the left ventricle during isovolumetric contraction. It is measured before aortic valve opening and thus before any change in left atrial pressure.

It is obtained using pulsed wave Doppler in apical four chambers. The maximal rise in pressure is obtained and computed from the time interval between 1 and 3 m/s (Fig. 10.5).

While attractive, this indice is often limited by the difficulty to obtain a mitral regurgitant flow trace good enough for performing these measurements.

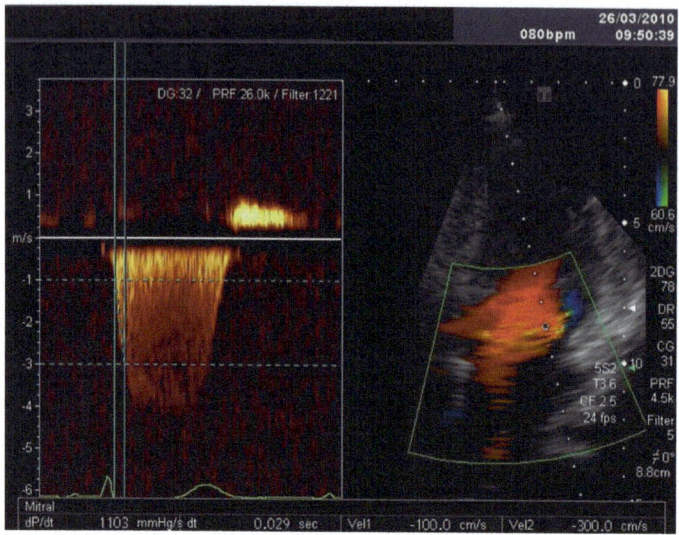

FIGURE 10.5 Maximal dP/dT from mitral regurgitant jet. Obtained from apical 4-chamber view

10.3.4 Global Longitudinal Strain by Speckle Tracking

Speckle tracking characterizes a method in which ultrasound echoes, or speckles, are tracked throughout the cardiac cycle. It allows to follow and quantify cardiac muscle wall motion. Cardiac motion is occurring in three directions: circumferential (rotational in heart short axis), radial (inward in heart short axis), and longitudinal (in LV long axis). Strain defines the difference in final length of a given heart segment relative to its resting length (L1–L0)/L0, expressed in percentage. Global longitudinal strain represents the longitudinal heart contraction obtained from averaging the longitudinal contraction of six myocardial segments in apical 4-chamber view (representing the septal, apical, and inferior left ventricular wall) (Fig. 10.6). It is a sensitive measurement of myocardial contractility.

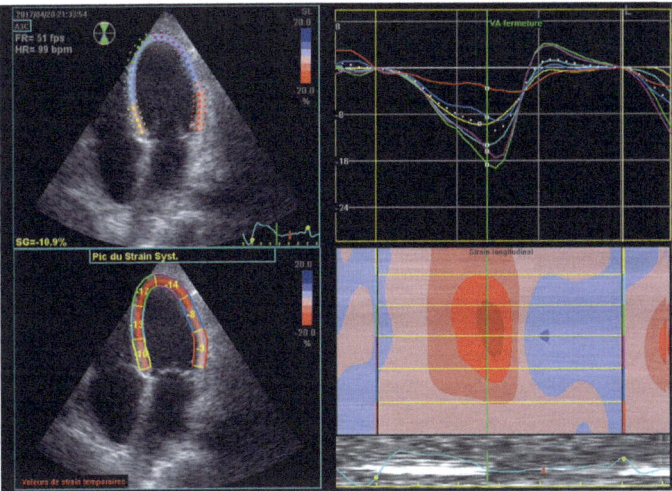

FIGURE 10.6 Global longitudinal strain. Obtained from apical 4-chamber view

Specific software, available on modern advanced echocardiographic devices, and also specific skills are required to measure global longitudinal strain. In addition, good apical views are required.

The advantage of this technique is that in integrates the movement of all parts of the left ventricle. While strain identifies subtle alterations in myocardial longitudinal contractility, this method does not evaluate the consequences of the altered contractility and hence does not indicate whether inotropic stimulation is indicated.

10.4 How to Use These Measurements in Practice

10.4.1 Cardiac Output and VTIao in Practice?

Beyond reliability of measurements, the most important aspect is how to interpret the measurements. Cardiac output is a variable that adapts to metabolic needs. Accordingly, a given value is seldom of marked relevance. It has to be confronted to clinical and biological indices of tissue perfusion. In a shocked patient, a high cardiac output is pathognomonic of distributive shock, while a low cardiac output is observed in the other types of shock.

Changes in VTIao, spontaneous or in response to therapy, are more relevant than changes in cardiac output. Indeed, changes in VTIao are not affected by errors in measuring LVOT diameter and, more importantly, are not affected by changes in heart rate and reflect more directly changes in stroke volume.

10.4.2   Evaluation of LV Contractility in Practice?

LV contractility is usually first evaluated by eyeball estimation of ejection fraction. When significant regional wall motion abnormalities are observed, measurement of ejection fraction by Simpson's method (2D and 4D), S wave tissue Doppler, or speckle tracking are preferred. Measurements of dP/dT_{max} can be useful whenever available. Combining several measurements is interesting, especially when regional wall motion abnormalities are detected. In the presence of significant valvular rejection, measurements of ejection fraction can be misleading, and the alternative methods should be preferred.

Suggested Readings

Bergenzaun L, Ohlin H, Gudmundsson P, Willenheimer R, Chew MS. Mitral annular plane systolic excursion (MAPSE) in shock: a valuable echocardiographic parameter in intensive care patients. Cardiovasc Ultrasound. 2013;11:16.

De Backer D, Cholley B, Vieillard-Baron A, Slama M, Vignon P. Hemodynamic monitoring using echocardiography in the critically ill. London: Springer; 2011.

Huang SJ, Ting I, Huang AM, Slama M, McLean AS. Longitudinal wall fractional shortening: an M-mode index based on mitral annular plane systolic excursion (MAPSE) that correlates and predicts left ventricular longitudinal strain (LVLS) in intensive care patients. Crit Care. 2017;21(1):292.

Orde SR, Pulido JN, Masaki M, Gillespie S, Spoon JN, Kane GC, et al. Outcome prediction in sepsis: speckle tracking echocardiography based assessment of myocardial function. Crit Care. 2014;18(4):R149.

Vieillard-Baron A, Charron C, Chergui K, Peyrouset O, Jardin F. Bedside echocardiographic evaluation of hemodynamics in sepsis: is a qualitative evaluation sufficient? Intensive Care Med. 2006;32(10):1547–52.

Chapter 11
LV Diastolic Function and PAOP

Anthony McLean

Elevation of left ventricular end-diastolic pressure (LVEDP) or left atrial pressure (LAP), of which the pulmonary artery pressure (PAOP) is a surrogate marker, occurs under a number of conditions, including left ventricular systolic dysfunction, diastolic dysfunction and a combination of the two, aortic valve dysfunction, and left ventricular outflow obstruction. Assessment of the LVEDP, or the LAP, which is nearly identical in the absence of significant mitral valve disease, is a primary objective in assessing the circulation. The echocardiographic parameters used to evaluate LAP are similar to those used for the assessment of diastolic dysfunction (DD) since the latter causes elevation of the former. A critical care physician is less concerned with the relative contributions of left ventricular systolic and diastolic dysfunction to an elevated LAP and more with what is the actual pressure so as to manipulate therapy accordingly.

A. McLean (✉)
Department of Intensive Care Medicine, Nepean Hospital, University of Sydney, Sydney, NSW, Australia
e-mail: anthony.mclean@sydney.edu.au

© Springer Nature Switzerland AG 2020
M. Slama (ed.), *Echocardiography in ICU*,
https://doi.org/10.1007/978-3-030-32219-9_11

11.1   Left Atrial Pressure (LAP)/Pulmonary Artery Occlusive Pressure (PAOP)

The parameters required to assess LAP in patients with a normal LVEF are mitral inflow E/A ratio, average E/e', tricuspid regurgitant velocity, and left atrial volume. Other parameters, such as mitral E deceleration time and pulmonary venous wave form, can still contribute on occasions (Fig. 11.1).

Box 11.1

PAOP and then E/A or E/e' ratios do not predict fluid responsiveness and should not be used to decide fluid expansion.

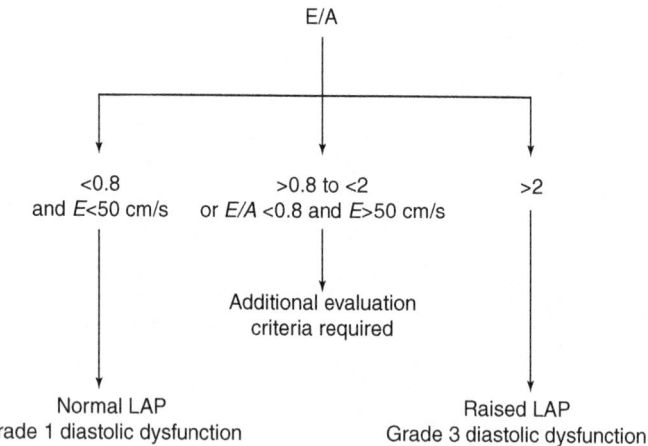

Figure 11.1 Assessment of LAP (left atrial pressure) = PAOP (pulmonary artery occlusive pressure)

Box 11.2

PAOP and then *E/A* or *E/e'* ratios should be used to assess the tolerance of fluid expansion.

Box 11.3

PAOP and then *E/A* ratios are used as a surrogate of wedge pressure to discriminate ARDS and hemodynamic pulmonary edema.

Box 11.4

E/A velocity measurements:

The sampling box of the pulse wave Doppler is placed at the tips of the mitral leaflets in diastole. The E velocity is measured and E/A ratio calculated.

Box 11.5   Assessment of Left Atrial Pressure (LAP) or Pulmonary Artery Occlusive Pressure (PAOP)

Additional criteria for high LAP/PAOP (at least two of them):

1. *Average E/e''* (mitral *E* inflow velocity is divided by the average of the medial and lateral mitral *e'* measurements).
   E/e' > 15 high LAP/PAOP (E/e' < 6 low or normal LAP/PAOP).
2. *Tricuspid regurgitant velocity > 2.8 m/s.*
3. *LA volume index > 34 ml/m2.*

11.2   Left Ventricular Diastolic Function

In ICU it is challenging to apply ASE recommendations to assess left ventricular diastolic function due to the fact that the impairment of relaxation could be, or not be, associated with high LV filling pressure. A recent work suggests a medial e'/s' ratio <0.86 may be a good indicator of diastolic dysfunction in critically ill patients (Nepean ratio). Also, dilatation of the left atrium does not occur acutely.

Box 11.6

Assessment of left ventricular relaxation:
- E' lateral <10 cm/s and/or E' septal <8 cm/s.
- Dilation of the left atrium >34 ml/m².
- Absence of mitral calcification or segmental dysfunction involving lateral or septal wall.

Multiple Choice Questions

1. Regarding the E/A ratio:

    A. E/A ratio >2 is usually associated with low PAOP.
    B. E/A ratio >2 is most of the time associated with high PAOP.
    C. In a patient with suspicion of pulmonary edema, $E/e' > 15$ confirms a hemodynamic cause.
    D. Pulmonary hypertension is always associated with high E/e' ratio.
    Answers: B, C

2. In a patient with suspected ARDS:
    A. E/A ratio is usually >2.
    B. Left atrium is enlarged.
    C. E/e' ratio is always <6.
    D. E/e' is usually <15.
    E. E/e' may be >15 when associated with volume overload.
    Answers: D, E

Further Readings

Clancy DJ, Slama M, Huang S, et al. Detecting impaired myocardial relaxation in sepsis with a novel tissue Doppler parameter (septal e′/s′). Crit Care. 2017;21:175–84.

Nagueh SF, Simseth OA, Appleton CP, et al. Recommendations for the evaluation of left ventricular diastolic function by echocardiography. J Am Soc Echocardiogr. 2016;29:277–314.

Chapter 12
Right Ventricular Function

Antoine Vieillard-Baron

In many situations encountered in the ICU, an RV failure may be the main mechanism of shock and then should be systematically detected by echocardiography. Five echo parameters are mandatory, and some are optional (Figs. 12.1, 12.2, and 12.3).

Electronic Supplementary Material   The online version of this chapter (https://doi.org/10.1007/978-3-030-32219-9_12) contains supplementary material, which is available to authorized users.

A. Vieillard-Baron (✉)
Surgical and Medical ICU, University Hospital Ambroise Paré, APHP, Boulogne-Billancourt, France
e-mail: antoine.vieillard-baron@aphp.fr

© Springer Nature Switzerland AG 2020
M. Slama (ed.), *Echocardiography in ICU*,
https://doi.org/10.1007/978-3-030-32219-9_12

140   A. Vieillard-Baron

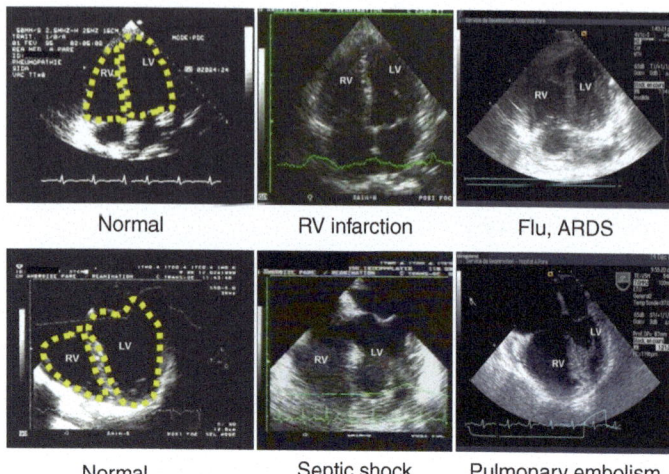

| Normal | RV infarction | Flu, ARDS |

| Normal | Septic shock | Pulmonary embolism |

FIGURE 12.1 The ratio between the end-diastolic area of the RV and the LV (RV/LV EDA) to evaluate RV size. It has to be calculated or visually evaluated on a four-chamber view (apical by TTE or mid-esophageal at 0° by TEE). RV is nondilated when the ratio is ≤0.6 and the RV keeps its normal triangular shape. The RV is moderately dilated when the ratio is >0.6 and <1. The RV is severely dilated when the ratio is >1 (the RV is bigger than the LV). When dilated, the RV loses its triangular shape. In case of left ventricular dilation, large RV is diagnosed using right ventricular area >12 cm²/m²

| Pulmonary embolism | ARDS Mechanical |
| Spontaneous ventilation | ventilation |

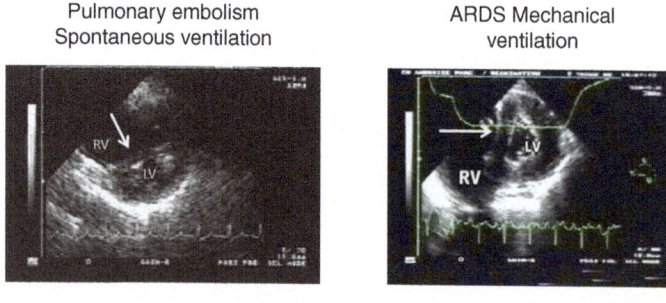

FIGURE 12.2 The movement of the interventricular septum on a short axis (parasternal or transgastric) to look for a paradoxical septal motion. During diastole, it reflects a huge RV diastolic overload, while in end systole an RV systolic overload. An example by TTE and TEE

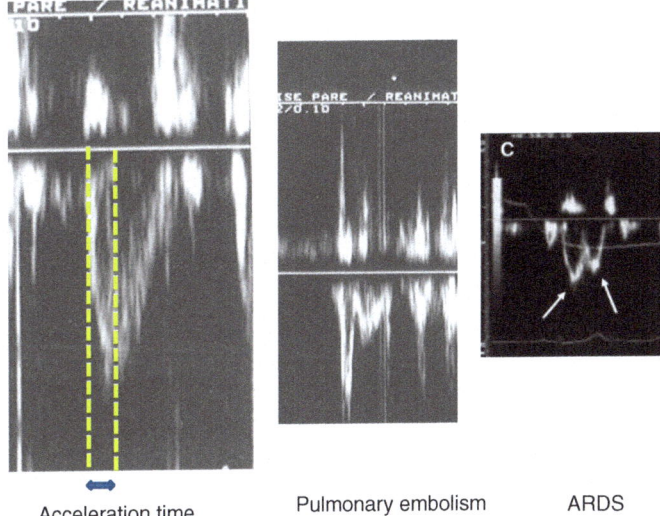

Acceleration time   Pulmonary embolism   ARDS

FIGURE 12.3 The acceleration time of the RV ejection flow. It is measured using the pulsed-wave Doppler in a parasternal short-axis view (TTE) or upper esophageal view at 0° (TEE). A value below 100 ms is very suggestive of a significant pulmonary hypertension. When associated with a biphasic pattern, it suggests an obstruction (proximal in pulmonary embolism or distal in ARDS) of the pulmonary circulation

---

Box 12.1 Five Mandated Parameters to Assess RV Function

The five required parameters:
- The ratio between the end-diastolic area of the RV and the LV (RV/LV EDA) to evaluate RV size
- The movement of the interventricular septum on a short axis (parasternal or transgastric) to look for a paradoxical septal motion
- The respiratory variations of the RV ejection flow
- The collapsibility index of the superior vena cava
- The tricuspid regurgitation flow and/or the acceleration time of the RV ejection flow

Box 12.2 Acute or Chronic Cor Pulmonale?

The association of an RV dilatation with a paradoxical septal motion defines cor pulmonale, which is acute according to the following:

1. Clinical context
2. RV free wall thickness <5 mm
3. Systolic pulmonary artery pressure (SPAP) <60 mmHg. SPAP is calculated using the simplified Bernoulli equation as SPAP = $4 \times V^2$ + POD, where V is the maximal velocity of the tricuspid regurgitation using the continuous wave Doppler

Many other parameters have been proposed, from the simplest to the more "complicated," most of them with limitations related either to technical issues or to a low value for practical application in critically ill patients (Table 12.1). Briefly, the shortening of the RV long axis may be evaluated by measuring the degree of displacement or the speed of displacement of the lateral part of the tricuspid annulus. The former requires combining 2D and M-mode to measure the

TABLE 12.1 The optional parameters of RV systolic function

Parameters	Abnormal value
TAPSE	<16 mm
S' wave	<11.5 cm/s
FAC	<35%
Strain	> −20%
dP/dt	<400 mmHg/s

TAPSE: tricuspid annular plan systolic excursion, FAC: fractional area contraction; dP/dt is the pressure gradient generated by the right ventricle during the early systole; it is calculated using the tricuspid regurgitation

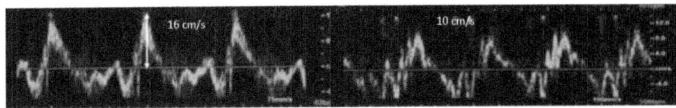

FIGURE 12.4 Tissue Doppler imaging (TDI) to measure the maximal velocity during systole (S′ wave)

tricuspid annular plan systolic excursion (TAPSE). The latter requires using tissue Doppler imaging (TDI) to measure the maximal velocity during systole (S′ wave) (Fig. 12.4). Both cannot be obtained using the TEE. The RV fractional area contraction is obtained from four cavities (TTE or TEE) and is calculated as the end-diastolic area minus the end-systolic area/the end-diastolic area. Recently, RV longitudinal strain has also been proposed for evaluating RV function but is not now recommended at the bedside in the ICU.

Multiple Choice Questions

1. In case of acute cor pulmonale, echocardiography may visualize:

   A. An RV dilatation.
   B. The absence of respiratory variation of the RV ejection flow.
   C. A systolic pulmonary artery pressure above 70 mmHg.
   D. A complete collapse of the SVC during insufflation.
   E. A paradoxical septal motion.
   Answers: A, E

2. Among the following parameters, which are the ones that were proposed to evaluate RV systolic function?

   A. MAPSE.
   B. TAPSE.
   C. dP/dt on the pulmonary regurgitation.
   D. dP/dt on the tricuspid regurgitation.
   E. FAC.
   Answers: B, D, E

3. Concerning RV ejection flow, which assertions are true?

   A. A biphasic pattern is pathognomonic of a massive pulmonary embolism.
   B. An acceleration time below 100 ms is very suggestive of pulmonary hypertension.
   C. A biphasic pattern is a sign of an obstruction of the pulmonary circulation.
   D. An acceleration time below 100 ms is a normal value.
   E. Evaluation of the RV ejection flow requires using the continuous wave Doppler.

   Answers: B, C

Suggested Readings

Jardin F, Vieillard-Baron A. Monitoring f right-sided heart function. Curr Opin Crit Care. 2005;11:271–9.

Rudski LG, Lai WW, Afilalo J, et al. Guidelines for the echocardiographic assessment of the right heart in adults: a report from the American society of echocardiography endorsed by the European association of echocardiography, a registered branch of the European society of cardiology, and the Canadian society of echocardiography. J Am Soc Echocariogr. 2010;23:685–713.

Vieillard-Baron A, Naeije R, Haddad F, et al. Diagnostic workup, etiologies and management of acute right ventricle failure. Intensive Care Med. 2018;44(6):774–90.

Vieillard-Baron A. Assessment of right ventricular function. Curr Opin Crit Care. 2009;15:254–60.

Chapter 13
Pulmonary Artery Pressures

Daniel De Backer

Pulmonary hypertension is a common finding in critically ill patients; it can occur as a result of increased pulmonary artery resistance (in most cases in capillaries but can also be due to the obstruction of pulmonary artery vessels and even sometimes in pulmonary veins) or an increase in left atrial pressures. Importantly, even though often associated with signs of right ventricular dysfunction, right ventricular function can be preserved in the face of moderate pulmonary hypertension. On the other hand, right ventricular function can be altered in the absence of pulmonary hypertension (i.e., right ventricular myocardial infarction), and measurements

D. De Backer (✉)
Department of Intensive Care, CHIREC Hospitals, Université Libre de Bruxelles, Brussels, Belgium
e-mail: ddebacke@ulb.ac.be

© Springer Nature Switzerland AG 2020
M. Slama (ed.), *Echocardiography in ICU*,
https://doi.org/10.1007/978-3-030-32219-9_13

of pulmonary artery pressures are useful in order to identify the cause of right ventricular dysfunction. Accordingly, the estimation of pulmonary artery pressure is important and can be performed by different methods in critically ill patients (Table 13.1).

TABLE 13.1 Measurements of pulmonary artery pressure

Measurement	TTE views	TEE views	Interpretation
Tricuspid regurgitation (PAPsyst)	A4C or PSA	Long axis ME or deep transgastric (often off angle)	Normal 25–30 mmHg HTAP >35 mmHg
Pulmonary valve regurgitation (PAPmean)	PSA or subxyphoidal	Long axis UE or transgastric	Normal 15–20 mmHg HTAP >25 mmHg
Pulmonary valve regurgitation (PAPdiast)	PSA or subxyphoidal	Long axis UE or transgastric	Normal 10–15 mmHg HTAP >20 mmHg
Pulmonary artery acceleration time	PSA or subxyphoidal	Long axis UE or transgastric	Normal >100 ms HTAP <90 ms
Pulmonary artery acceleration morphology	PSA or subxyphoidal	Long axis UE or transgastric	Biphasic flow suggestive of severe pulmonary hypertension

PAPsyst systolic pulmonary artery pressure, *PAPmean* mean pulmonary artery pressure, *PAPdiast* diastolic pulmonary artery pressure, *A4C* apical four-chamber view, *PSA* parasternal short axis, *ME* mid esophageal, *UE* upper esophageal, *HTAP* pulmonary hypertension See text for formulas

13.1   Systolic Pulmonary Artery Pressure from Tricuspid Regurgitant Jet

Systolic pulmonary artery pressure is best estimated from tricuspid regurgitant flow (Fig. 13.1). According to the simplified Bernouilli equation, systolic pulmonary artery pressure can be calculated as 4 × (tricuspid regurgitant jet peak velocity)^2 + right atrial pressure (RAP). Pulmonary artery pressure measurements are more reliable when RAP is measured using a central venous catheter. Alternatively, RAP can be semi-quantitatively estimated using inferior vena cava size and its variability along the respiratory cycle.

Tricuspid regurgitant flow should be obtained from apical four chambers or in parasternal short axis (with angulation of the probe to the upper part of thorax) using color Doppler for the localization of tricuspid regurgitant flow and continuous Doppler for its quantification. A good signal envelope is required, and every effort should be made to minimize the angle between the jet and the beam (Fig. 13.1).

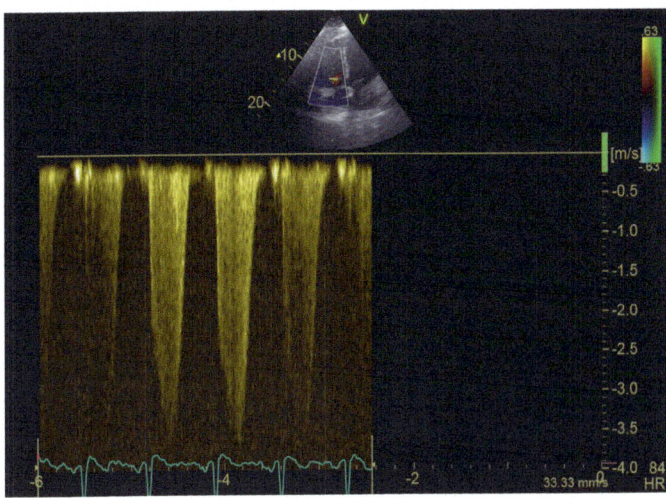

FIGURE 13.1 Tricuspid regurgitant flow. The tricuspid maximal velocity is at 3.5 m/s. Accordingly, PAPs was 49 mmHg + RAP

13.2   Mean and Diastolic Pulmonary Artery Pressures from Pulmonary Valve Regurgitant Jet

Mean and diastolic pulmonary artery pressures can be estimated from pulmonary valve regurgitation jet (Fig. 13.2). The mean and diastolic pulmonary artery pressures are estimated from the peak and end-diastolic velocities of regurgitant jet, respectively (Fig. 13.2). According to the simplified Bernouilli equation, the mean pulmonary artery pressure is 4 × (pulmonary regurgitant peak velocity)^2 + RAP and pulmonary artery diastolic pressure 4 × (pulmonary regurgitant end-diastolic velocity)^2 + RAP.

Pulmonary valve regurgitant flow should be obtained from parasternal short axis (with angulation of the probe to the

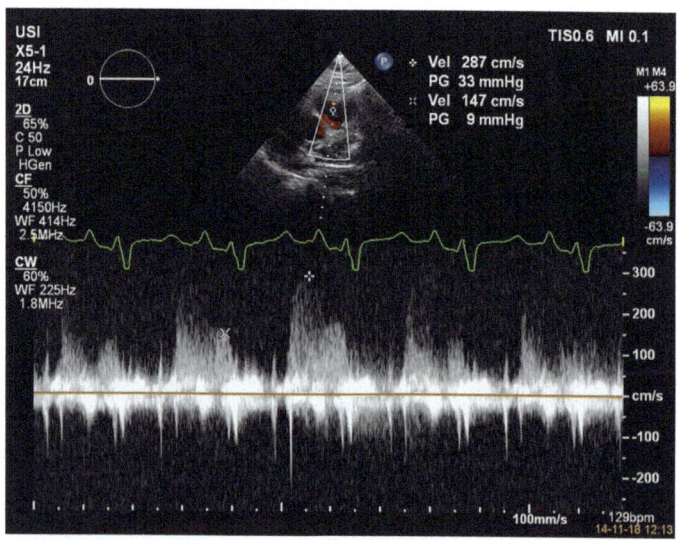

FIGURE 13.2 Pulmonary valve regurgitant flow. The maximal velocity was 2.87 m/s, suggesting a PAPmean at 33 mmHg + RAP. The end diastolic velocity was 1.47 m/s, suggesting a PAPdiast at 9 mmHg + RAP

upper part of thorax) or subxyphoidal view using color Doppler for the localization of pulmonary regurgitant flow and continuous Doppler for its quantification.

Unfortunately, pulmonary valve regurgitation is inconstantly observed, even though more frequent in patient with pulmonary hypertension, admittedly.

13.3   Acceleration and Morphology of Pulmonary Artery Flow

Pulmonary artery flow morphology is altered in pulmonary hypertension. Pulmonary acceleration time can be used to estimate pulmonary artery pressure (Fig. 13.3). The rise in velocity is sharper in pulmonary hypertension. Formulas exist to compute PAPsyst from acceleration time, but these are infrequently used. Estimation of acceleration time requires

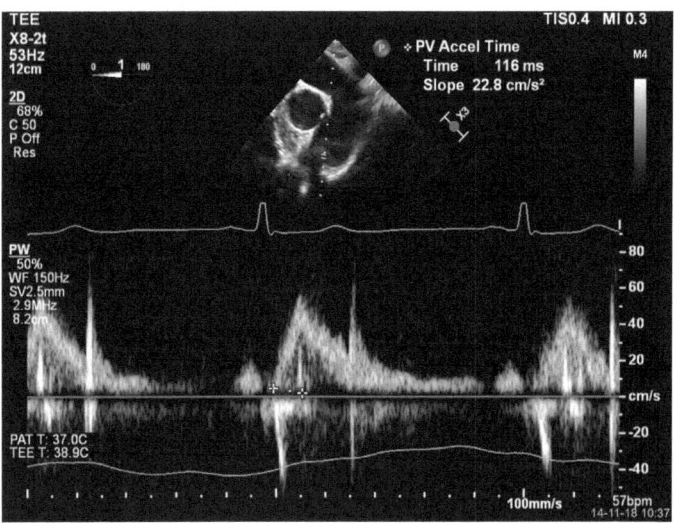

FIGURE 13.3 Pulmonary artery acceleration time measured from TEE view of pulmonary edema (pulmonary flow is positive). Acceleration time was recorded at 116 ms, suggesting a normal PAP. Please also note the normal pattern of pulmonary artery velocities

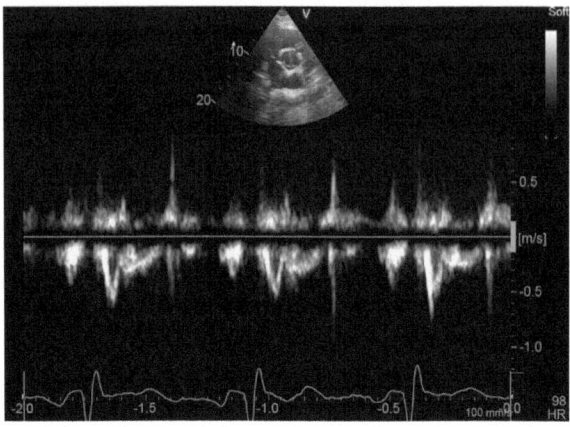

FIGURE 13.4 Typical biphasic pulmonary artery flow

that heart rate is between 60 and 100–120 bpm. In severe cases, a biphasic flow can be observed (Fig. 13.4).

Pulmonary artery flow is recorded in parasternal short axis or subxyphoidal views, applying pulse wave Doppler with a sampling volume just distal to the pulmonary valve.

Suggested Readings

De Backer D, Cholley BP, Slama M, Vieillard-Baron A, Vignon P. Hemodynamic monitoring using echocardiography in the critically ill. New York: Springer; 2011.

Jardin F, Dubourg O, Bourdarias JP. Echocardiographic pattern of acute cor pulmonale. Chest. 1997;111(1):209–17.

Rudski LG, Lai WW, Afilalo J, Hua L, Handschumacher MD, Chandrasekaran K, et al. Guidelines for the echocardiographic assessment of the right heart in adults: a report from the American Society of Echocardiography endorsed by the European Association of Echocardiography, a registered branch of the European Society of Cardiology, and the Canadian Society of Echocardiography. J Am Soc Echocardiogr. 2010;23(7):685–713.

Part V
Shocks

Chapter 14
Hypovolemic Shock

Michel Slama

14.1 Introduction

Hypovolemic shock is usually easy to recognize; nevertheless, there are many circumstances for which hypovolemia is hard to be diagnosed. Then we provide useful algorithms that may help to decide to do a volume expansion (Figs. 14.1 and 14.2).

M. Slama (✉)
Medical ICU, CHU Sud, Amiens, France
e-mail: slama.michel@chu-amiens.fr

© Springer Nature Switzerland AG 2020   153
M. Slama (ed.), *Echocardiography in ICU*,
https://doi.org/10.1007/978-3-030-32219-9_14

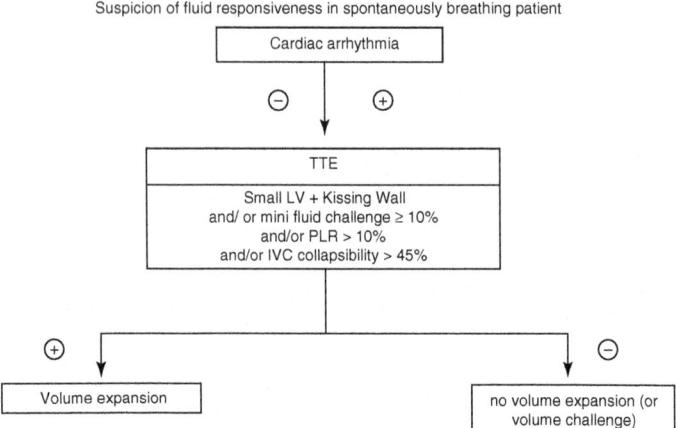

FIGURE 14.1 Algorithm to assess fluid responsiveness in spontaneously breathing patients

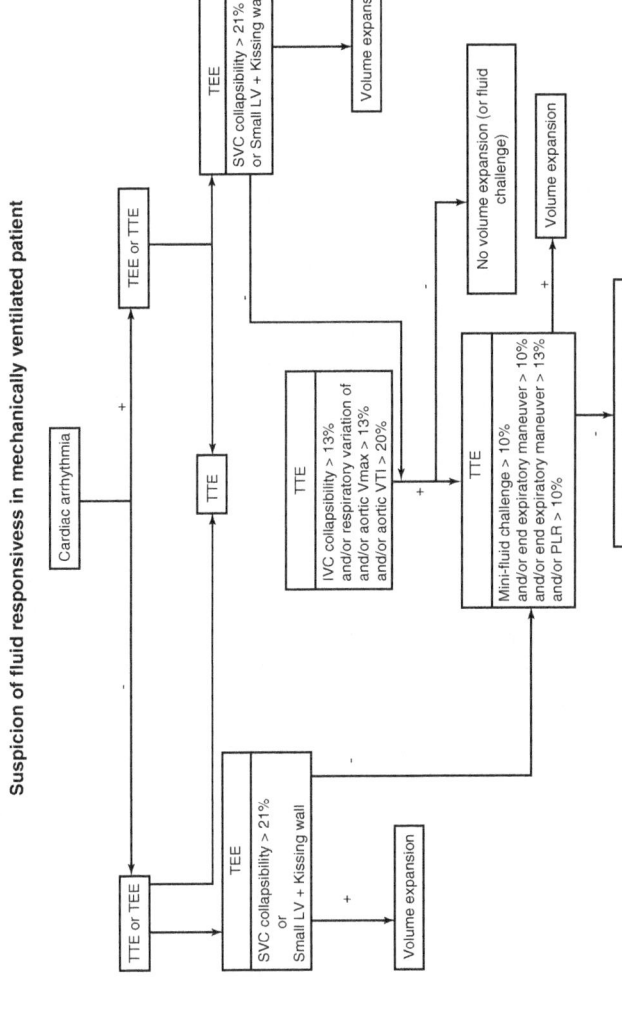

FIGURE 14.2 Algorithm to assess fluid responsivess in patients under mechanical ventilation

Chapter 15
Cardiogenic Shock

Anthony McLean

15.1 Introduction

In this chapter, two algorithms to support clinicians in how to manage patients with cardiogenic shock are supplied.

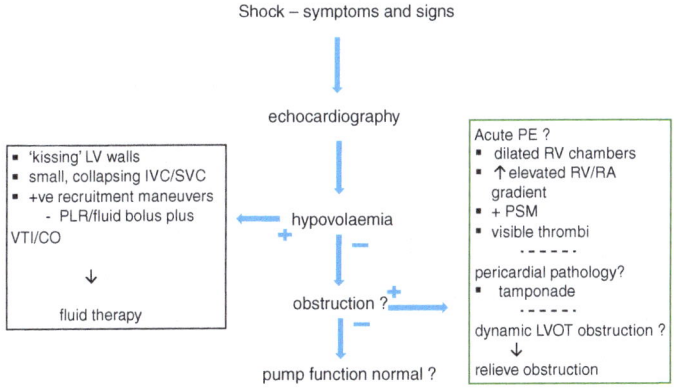

A. McLean (✉)
Department of Intensive Care Medicine, Nepean Hospital,
University of Sydney, Sydney, NSW, Australia
e-mail: anthony.mclean@sydney.edu.au

© Springer Nature Switzerland AG 2020   157
M. Slama (ed.), *Echocardiography in ICU*,
https://doi.org/10.1007/978-3-030-32219-9_15

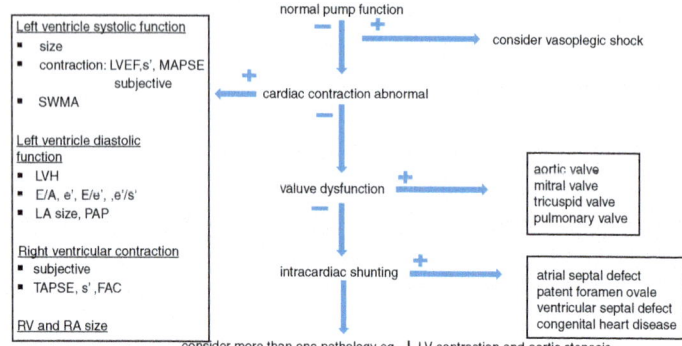

Left ventricle systolic function
- size
- contraction: LVEF,s', MAPSE subjective
- SWMA

Left ventricle diastolic function
- LVH
- E/A, e', E/e', ,e'/s'
- LA size, PAP

Right ventricular contraction
- subjective
- TAPSE, s' ,FAC

RV and RA size

normal pump function

consider vasoplegic shock

cardiac contraction abnormal

valuve dysfunction

aortic valve
mitral valve
tricuspid valve
pulmonary valve

intracardiac shunting

atrial septal defect
patent foramen ovale
ventricular septal defect
congenital heart disease

consider more than one pathology eg. ↓ LV contraction and aortic stenosis

Chapter 16
Septic Shock

Paul H. Mayo

This algorithm helps the clinician to manage patients with septic shock.

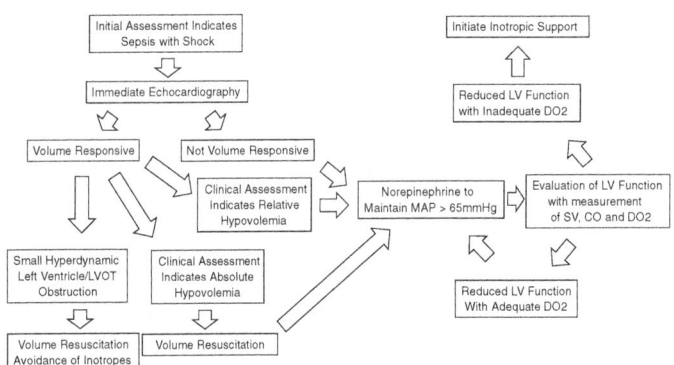

P. H. Mayo (✉)
Division Pulmonary, Critical Care, and Sleep Medicine, Northwell
Health, New York, NY, USA
e-mail: pmayo@northwell.edu

© Springer Nature Switzerland AG 2020
M. Slama (ed.), *Echocardiography in ICU*,
https://doi.org/10.1007/978-3-030-32219-9_16

Part VI
Respiratory Failures

Chapter 17
Respiratory Failure

Michel Slama

In this chapter, we provide *deux algorythme* to manage patients with respiratory failure: (1) "white chest X-ray" and (2) "black chest X-ray."

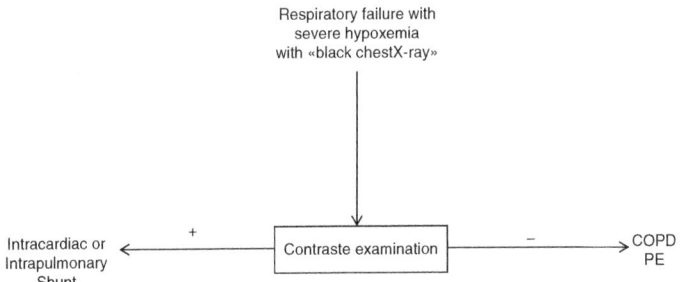

M. Slama (✉)
Medical ICU, CHU Sud, Amiens, France
e-mail: slama.michel@chu-amiens.fr

© Springer Nature Switzerland AG 2020
M. Slama (ed.), *Echocardiography in ICU*,
https://doi.org/10.1007/978-3-030-32219-9_17

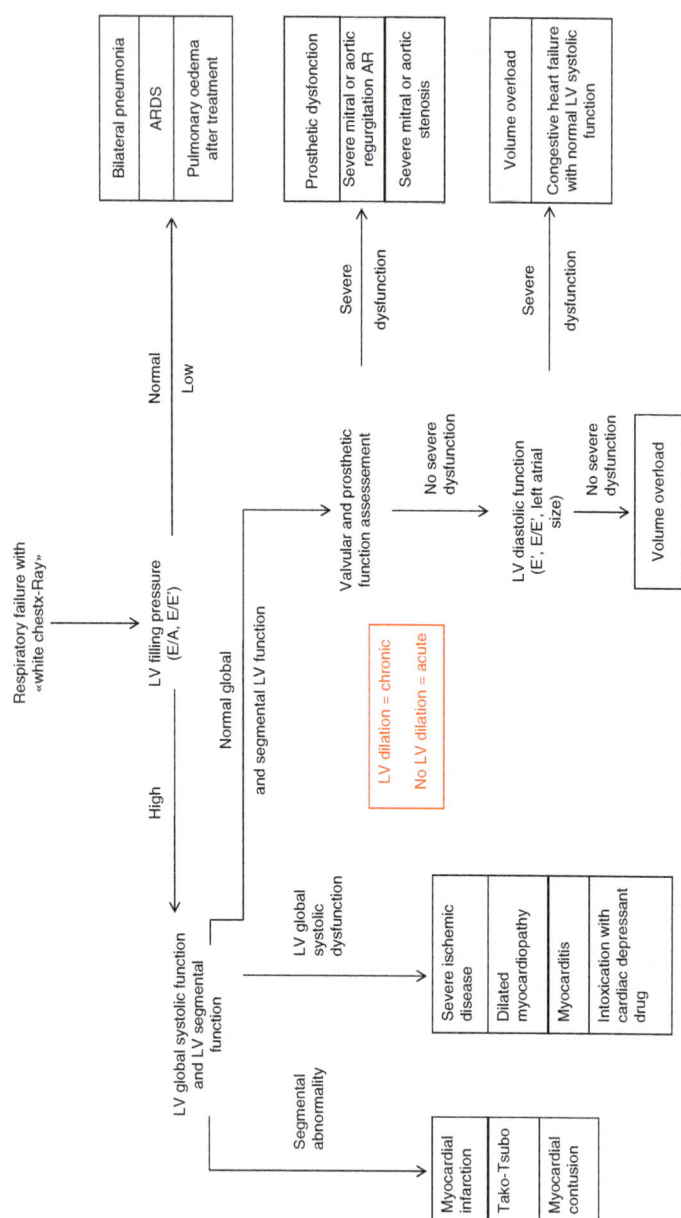

Chapter 18
Right to Left Shunt

Paul H. Mayo

A variety of critical illnesses are associated with the elevation of right-sided cardiac pressures. When this occurs, the patient with a patent foramen ovale (PFO) may develop a right-to-left shunt. Given that at least 20% of the normal population has a potentially patent PFO, intracardiac shunt is always a concern in the critically ill patient with severe hypoxemic respiratory failure who is on ventilatory support; the presence of a right-to-left shunt may contribute to hypoxemia, beyond which is caused by the primary lung disease. Echocardiography has immediate application for the detection of right-to-left intracardiac shunt in this clinical situation.

P. H. Mayo (✉)
Division Pulmonary, Critical Care, and Sleep Medicine,
Northwell Health, New York, NY, USA
e-mail: pmayo@northwell.edu

© Springer Nature Switzerland AG 2020
M. Slama (ed.), *Echocardiography in ICU*,
https://doi.org/10.1007/978-3-030-32219-9_18

How to Perform ASC Injection

1. A 10 cc syringe is filled with 9 cc normal saline and 1 cc air.
2. The saline syringe and second empty syringe are attached to a three-way stopcock
3. The saline is agitated vigorously by manually pumping it back and forth between the two syringes. This forms a suspension of microbubbles that constitutes the ASC.
4. The suspension should appear opaque, if adequately agitated between the two syringes.
5. The ACS is injected as rapidly as possible while simultaneously imaging the heart real time.
6. The preferred injection site is through the femoral vein, although adequate opacification of the right atrium can be achieved from sites in the arm or through a central line positioned in the superior vena cava.
7. With TTE, the subcostal, the apical four-chamber view, or the short-axis view of the base of the heart is used to visualize the right and left atrium. Following intravenous injection of ASC into the right atrium, identification of ASC in the left atrium constitutes evidence for a right-to-left shunt.
8. With transesophageal echocardiography, the bicaval view or the biatrial view at $0°$ is used for identification of right-to-left ACS transfer.

Pitfalls in the Detection of Right-to-Left Shunt

1. Color Doppler is not a reliable means of detecting right-to-left shunt through a PFO.
2. Detection of right-to-left shunt with ACS using TTE requires good image quality. Patient-specific factors, hyperinflation, and difficulty with positioning the critically ill patient may combine to degrade image quality. TEE is always an option.
3. Inflow from the inferior vena cava is preferentially directed toward the interatrial septum. If the ACS

enters via the superior vena cava, the IVC inflow may block ACS from reaching the septum. This may result in a false negative study. Femoral venous injection is preferred but not required.

4. For intravenous ACS to detect a right to left shunt, RA pressure must be higher than LA pressure. However, a patent PFO without right-to-left shunt is not of immediate concern to the intensivist, who is primarily concerned with the contribution that a PFO might have to hypoxemia. This only occurs when there is a right-to-left shunt.

5. There is no validated means of quantitating the severity of right-to-left shunt detected with ACS. The severity of shunt is determined by the pressure gradient between the two atria and the size of the atrial defect. The intensivist may make a qualitative estimate of the severity based on the number of bubbles that are visualized.

6. Spontaneous echo contrast may be mistaken for ASC by the inexperienced scanner.

7. Coughing transiently increases RA pressure, so coughing may be used as a provocative maneuver during ASC injection to detect a potentially patent PFO.

8. For the patients on ventilatory support without volitional cough capability, an increase in PEEP level or an inspiratory hold for the duration of the ASC injection may be used as a provocative maneuver to increase RA pressure in order to detect a patent PFO.

9. While the most common cause of right-to-left shunt detected with echocardiography is a patent PFO, the intensivist checks with 2-D echocardiography for rare causes of right-to-left shunt (ASD and VSD) and remains alert for the possibility of intrapulmonary shunt. The latter manifests with a delay of four or more cardiac cycles between ASC opacification of the RA and bubble detection in the LA. Where the timing is indeterminate (i.e., between three and four cardiac cycle delays), TEE is useful for direct observation of microbubbles exiting the pulmonary veins.

Clinical Implications of a Right-to-Left Shunt

1. While echocardiographic detection of a right-to-left shunt in the noncritically ill patient is used to evaluate for paradoxical embolism (e.g., cryptogenic stroke) or intrapulmonary shunt (e.g., hepatopulmonary syndrome with orthodeoxia), the intensivist is primarily interested in right-to-left shunt for its effect on oxygenation function.

2. The typical critically ill patient may or may not have a preexisting disease that has resulted in elevated right heart pressure (e.g., pulmonary arterial hypertension) that is combined with an acute process that requires positive pressure ventilatory support for severe hypoxemic respiratory failure, such as ARDS. Positive pressure ventilation and any underlying disease increase right-sided pressures, thereby opening the PFO with exacerbation of the hypoxemia.

3. In this situation, the MICU team takes action to reduce right-sided pressures in order to reduce the right-to-left shunt. These may include:

   (a) Reducing PEEP and cycling pressures of the ventilator cognizant of the possibility that this may result in hypercapnia and worsening hypoxemia, both of which may increase right ventricular (RV) afterload by increasing pulmonary artery pressure.

   (b) Considering the use of pulmonary vasodilators such as inhaled nitric oxide.

   (c) Considering the use of diuretic therapy to improve RV function.

   (d) Initiating early prone position ventilation, which is known to improve RV function.

   (e) Considering the use of ECMO to control hypercapnia and hypoxemia and their deleterious effects on pulmonary artery pressures.

(f) Considering the possibility of a prolonged recruit-ment maneuver with the possibility that recruit-ment of de-aerated lung will be accompanied by recruitment of vascular cross-sectional area and subsequent improvement in pulmonary artery pressures. The approach requires real-time moni-toring of hemodynamics and RV function with TEE, given the risk of precipitating severe acute cor pulmonale during the recruitment maneuver.

4. Using a closure device to block the intracardiac shunt is not indicated out of concern that closure of the PFO might result in augmentation of pulmonary artery blood with a deleterious effect on a compro-mised RV.

Suggested Readings

Bommer WJ, et al. The safety of contrast echocardiography: Report of the Committee on Contrast Echocardiography for the American Society of Echocardiography. J Am Coll Cardiol. 1984;3:6–13.

Konstadt SN, et al. Intraoperative detection of patent foramen ovale by transesophageal echocardiography. Anesthesiology. 1991;74:212–6.

Legras A, et al. Acute respiratory distress syndrome (ARDS)-associated acute cor pulmonale and patent foramen ovale: a mul-ticenter noninvasive hemodynamic study. Crit Care. 2015 Apr 17;19:174.

Mekontso-Dessap A, et al. Prevalence and prognosis of shunt-ing across patent foramen ovale during ARDS. Crit Care Med. 2010;38:1786–92.

Thanigaraj S, Valika A, Zajarias A, Lasala JM, Perez JE. Comparison of transthoracic versus transesophageal echocardiography for detection of right-to-left atrial shunting using agitated saline con-trast. Am J Cardiol. 2005;96:1007–10.

Part VII
Pathologies

Chapter 19
Pericardial Effusion and Tamponade

Paul H. Mayo

A pericardial effusion is a common finding on both TTE and TEE. Most are small and of no clinical consequence. A larger pericardial effusion raises the question as to etiology and whether there is hemodynamic consequence from pericardial tamponade. Echocardiography is useful to detect and characterize pericardial effusion, to identify findings consistent with tamponade, and to guide pericardiocentesis.

_____

Electronic Supplementary Material   The online version of this chapter (https://doi.org/10.1007/978-3-030-32219-9_19) contains supplementary material, which is available to authorized users.

_____

P. H. Mayo (✉)
Division Pulmonary, Critical Care, and Sleep Medicine, Northwell Health, New York, NY, USA
e-mail: pmayo@northwell.edu

© Springer Nature Switzerland AG 2020
M. Slama (ed.), *Echocardiography in ICU*,
https://doi.org/10.1007/978-3-030-32219-9_19

19.1   Identification of Pericardial Effusion

Pericardial fluid may be detected with TTE and TEE from many of the standard views, depending on its volume and distribution.

The parasternal long axis view is useful for detecting a small posterior pericardial effusion. With larger volumes of fluid, the effusion will distribute anterior to the right ventricular free wall.

The apical four-chamber view is useful for examining the movement of the right atrial free wall when there is pericardial fluid adjacent to it. This has utility when evaluating for pericardial tamponade.

The subcostal view is used to confirm the size of the pericardial effusion and to examine for cardiac chamber compression. It is the preferred view for the rapid assessment of hemopericardium during the evaluation of the trauma patient (Fig. 19.1).

> **Box 19.1 Recognizing Differences Between Pericardial and Pleural Effusion**
>
> A pleural effusion may be mistaken for a pericardial effusion, particularly from the parasternal long-axis view. The pleural effusion, which is identified as a relatively hypoechoic space posterior to the heart, distributes posterior to the descending aorta, whereas the *pericardial effusion distributes anterior to the descending aorta.*

19.2   Quantification of Pericardial Effusion

There is no widely accepted method for quantitating the size of a pericardial effusion. A pericardial effusion that is only visible in posterior position on the parasternal long-axis view

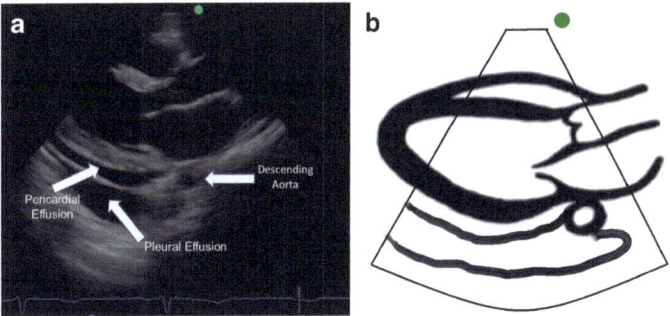

FIGURE 19.1 (**a**, **b**) Differentiation of pleural from pericardial effusion. In this parasternal long-axis view, the pleural effusion is positioned posterior to the descending aorta, whereas the cephalad extension of the pericardial effusion is anterior to the descending aorta

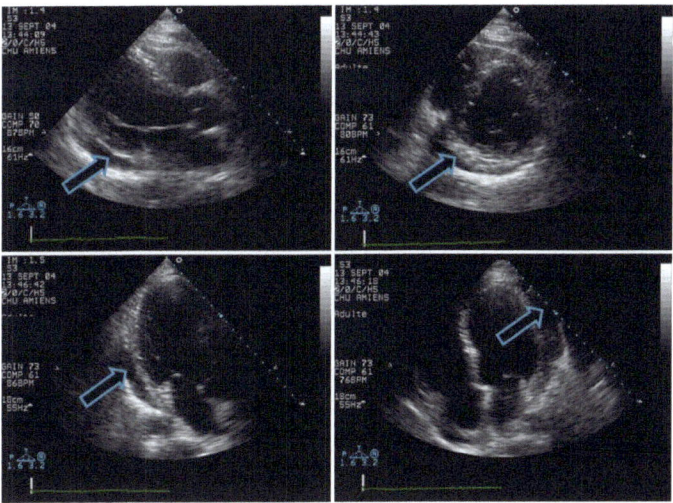

FIGURE 19.2 Echocardiographic images of small pericardial effusion

is reasonably classified as small. Once the pericardial effusion is circumferential, the distinction between moderate and large is subjective (Figs. 19.2 and 19.3).

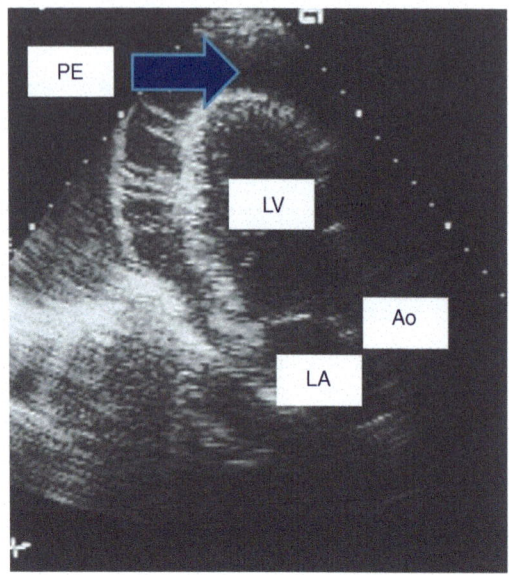

FIGURE 19.3 Echocardiographic image of pericardial effusion with strands

Box 19.2 Characterization of Pericardial Effusion

An anechoic pericardial effusion is likely to be a transu-date. The presence of increased echogenicity, stranding, septations, pericardial thickening, and/or masses are associated with exudative effusions related to infection or malignancy.

19.2.1   TEE for the Diagnosis of Pericardial Tamponade

If the patient has inadequate TTE views, TEE may be used to detect a pericardial effusion using views that are concomitant to standard TTE views. Small amounts of pericardial effusion are often identified adjacent to the great vessels in the high esophageal views. These are not visible on TTE and, unless associated with significant effusion elsewhere, are generally inconsequential.

In the postcardiac surgery patient who develops unexplained hypotension, a loculated pericardial effusion that compresses a cardiac chamber may have lethal outcome. These may not be visible on TTE due to their position or due to the poor image quality typical of the postcardiac surgery patient. Immediate TEE examination is required to identify this type of localized pericardial effusion, which, if present, may require immediate lifesaving surgical intervention.

Box 19.3 Fat or Effusion?

An anterior pericardial fat pad may be mistaken for a pericardial effusion. Pericardial fat has echogenic elements within it that move in synchrony with the cardiac pulsation.

19.3   Echocardiography Findings Consistent with Pericardial Tamponade

---

Box 19.4 Pericardial Tamponade Requires Clinical Evidence

There is no echocardiographic finding that is diagnostic of pericardial tamponade. The diagnosis of tamponade requires clinical evidence of hemodynamic compromise. Echocardiography serves to support the diagnosis but not to make it.

Box 19.5 2D Echocardiography in Pericardial Tamponade

Findings on 2-D echocardiography that support the diagnosis of pericardial tamponade:

1. Respirophasic variation of RV chamber size.
2. Nonphysiological movement of the right atrial free wall.
3. Nonphysiological movement of the right ventricular free wall.
4. Dilated IVC without respiratory changes.

1. *Respirophasic variation of RV chamber size* – this can be observed with 2-D imaging but can be documented with M-mode from the parasternal long-axis view with the M-mode cursor placed through the right ventricular (RV) free wall. Tamponade is associated with marked increases in RV dimension during inspiration (Fig. 19.4).
2. *Nonphysiological movement of the right atrial free wall* – inward movement of the RA free wall during systole in the presence of adjacent pericardial fluid represents chamber compression from the effusion. This supports the diagnosis of tamponade. Investigators have described a detailed measurement of the precise timing of the compression; these have limited clinical relevance (Figs. 19.5 and 19.6).
3. *Nonphysiological movement of the right ventricular free wall* – inward movement of the RV free wall during diastole in the presence of adjacent pericardial fluid represents chamber compression from the effusion (Figs. 19.7, 19.8, and 19.9).
4. IVC size and respirophasic variation – with pericardial tamponade, the IVC is dilated and lacks respirophasic size variation; this is due to impedance to RA inflow.

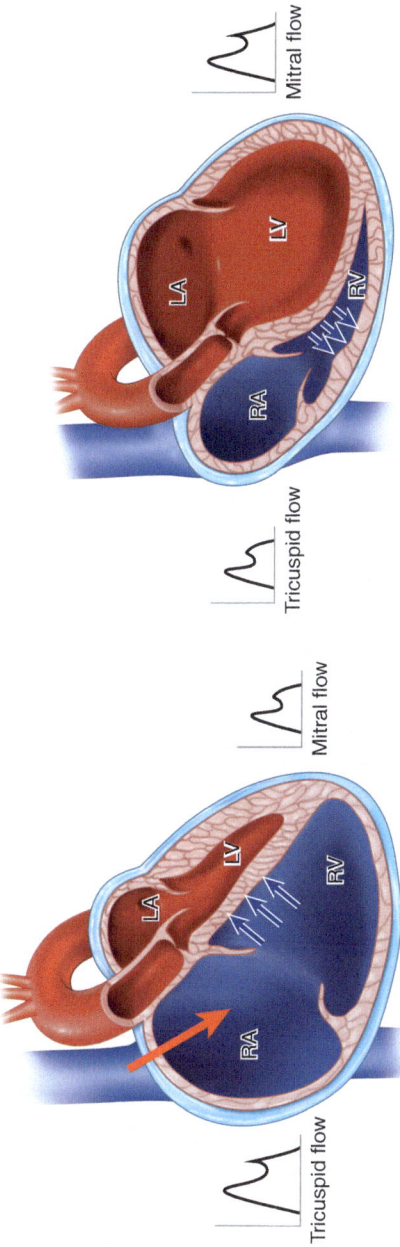

FIGURE 19.4 RV chamber variations (drawing) during inspiration (first figure) and expiratin (second figure) in spontaenously breathing patient. RA right atrium, RV right ventricle, LA left atrium, LV left ventricle

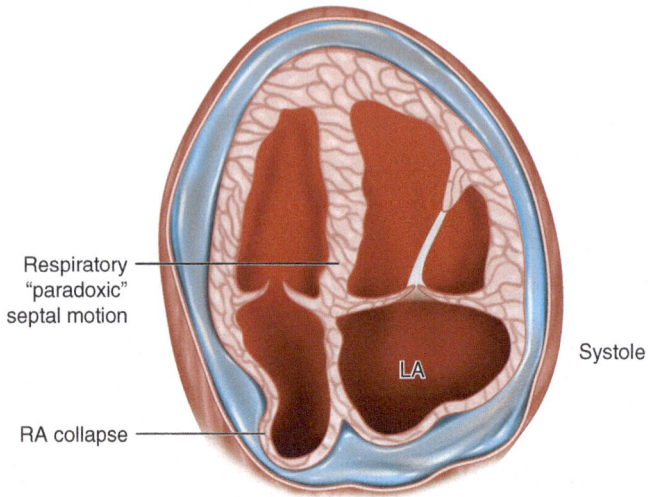

FIGURE 19.5 Diagram of nonphysiological movement of the right atrial free wall (drawing)

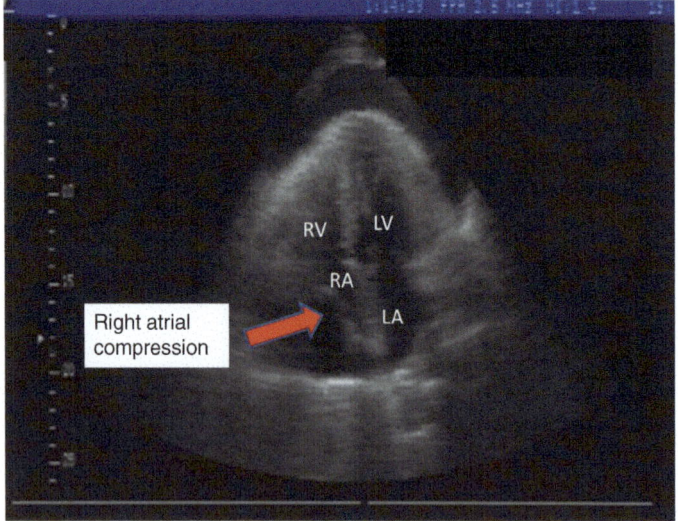

FIGURE 19.6 Echocardiographic image of nonphysiological movement of the right atrial free wall

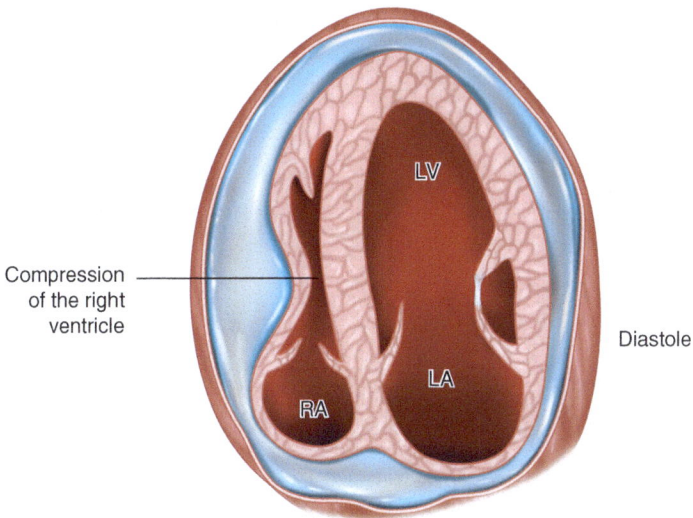

FIGURE 19.7 Diagram of nonphysiological movement of the right ventricular free wall (drawing)

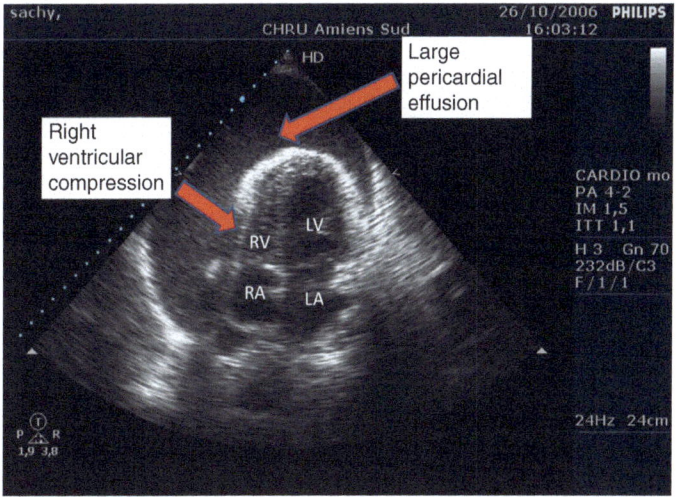

FIGURE 19.8 Diagram of nonphysiological movement of the right ventricular free wall. Compression of the RV

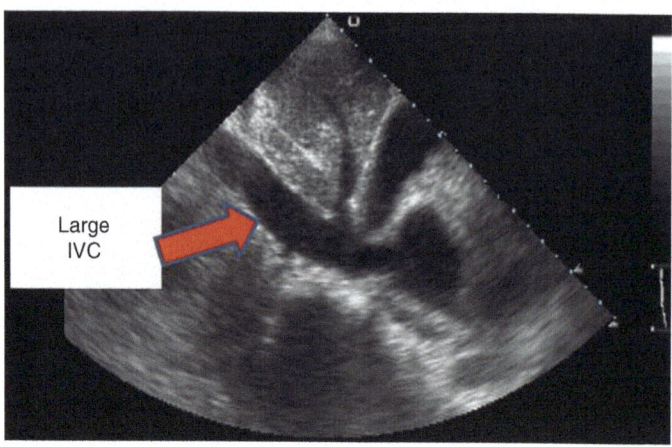

FIGURE 19.9 Large inferior vena cava

Box 19.6 Traps for the Diagnosis of Pericardial Tamponade

Both RA and RV compression are reduced when right-sided pressures are increased.

The presence of RV hypertrophy reduces compression effect, and the volume status of the patient may influence the degree of compression (Videos 19.1, 19.2, 19.3, 19.4, and 19.5. TTE examples of cardiac tamponade).

19.4   Findings on Doppler Echocardiography that Support the Diagnosis of Pericardial Tamponade

Respirophasic variation of peak mitral E-wave velocity – pericardial tamponade results in an increased respirophasic variation of stroke volume due to the augmentation of both serial and parallel interventricular interdependence. This is manifested by a reduced peak mitral E-wave velocity during inspiration compared to expiration. Greater than 30% variation of inspiratory and expiratory of peak mitral E-wave velocity is consistent with pericardial tamponade. Measurement of tricuspid valve peak E-wave velocity shows a reciprocal pattern of respirophasic variation. A more direct means of observing the respirophasic variation of SV that is characteristic of pericardial tamponade may be achieved by measuring respirophasic of the left ventricular outflow tract systolic velocity time integral peak velocity as a surrogate for SV. Alternatively, respirophasic variation of the brachial artery peak systolic velocity is a conveniently measured surrogate for SV variation. Respirophasic variation of SV may occur due to respirophasic variations of intrathoracic pressure that occur with airway obstruction or respiratory distress. This may result in a false positive diagnosis of pericardial tamponade in a patient who has distressed breathing, who has a pericardial effusion without pericardial tamponade (Fig. 19.10).

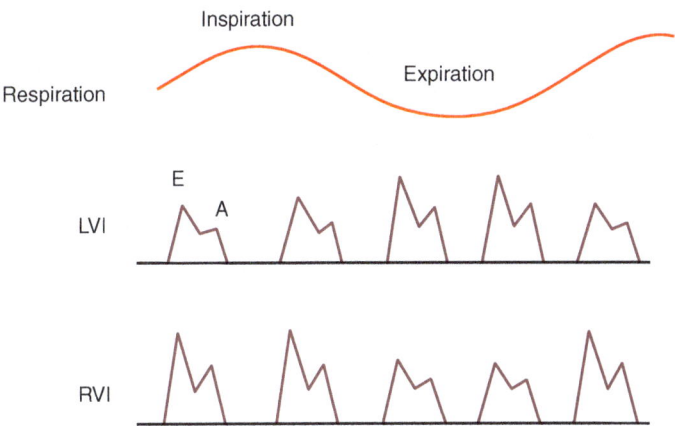

FIGURE 19.10 Respiratory variations of tricuspid and mitral flow (drawing)

19.5   Echocardiography for the Guidance of Pericardiocentesis (Fig. 19.11)

Box 19.7 Pericardiocentesis

1. Echocardiography is the preferred method for the safe guidance of pericardiocentesis.
2. The patient is scanned from the parasternal, apical, and subcostal views to identify a safe site, angle, and depth for needle insertion. The site is marked, the distance for needle insertion is measured (should be >10 mm for a safe puncture), and the angle for needle insertion is determined by the operator before sterile skin preparation. Following sterile preparation and a complete setup of all equipment, which includes the probe in a sterile sheath, the operator repeats the scan to confirm site, angle, and depth for needle penetration. The needle is inserted with free hand technique; real-time needle tip guidance is not necessary. Once fluid is aspirated, a wire is introduced over the needle with prompt needle removal. An appropriately sized catheter is then introduced over the wire. Catheter position can be confirmed with the injection of agitated saline contrast.
3. The most common site or needle insertion is from the apical position rather than the subcostal position. If the best site is from the parasternal position, color Doppler is used to identify and avoid the internal mammary artery. If there is concomitant interposed pleural effusion that blocks direct access to the pericardial fluid, it is advisable to first drain the pleural effusion, followed by the pericardiocentesis.

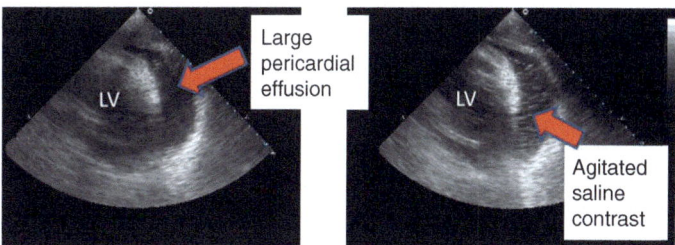

Large
pericardial
effusion

LV

LV

Agitated
saline
contrast

FIGURE 19.11 Large pericardial effusion drainage

Multiple Choice Questions

1. Regarding pericardial effusion:

   A. Is usually located in front of the right ventricle.
   B. Is usually located behind the left ventricle.
   C. From parasternal long-axis view is located behind the descending aorta.
   D. From parasternal long-axis view is located in front of the descending aorta.
   E. Could not be visualized after cardiac surgery using TTE.

   Answers: B, D, E

2. In a patient with shock, pericardial tamponade could be suspected when:

   A. There is a large pericardial effusion.
   B. There is a right atrial compression with pericardial effusion.
   C. There is right ventricular compression with pericardial effusion.
   D. There is large variations of tricuspid flow with large pericardial effusion.
   E. When there is large variations of aortic blood flow.

   Answers: A, B, C, D

Suggested Readings

1. Tsang TS, et al. Consecutive 1127 therapeutic echocardiographically guided pericardiocentesis: clinical profile, practice patterns, and outcomes spanning 21 years. Mayo Clin Proc. 2002;77:429–36.
2. Mekontso Dessap A, Chew MS. Cardiac tamponade. Inten Care Med. 2018;44:936–9.

Chapter 20
Echocardiography in ARDS

Antoine Vieillard-Baron

This chapter is finally no more than the combination and the summary of two others, i.e., heart–lung interactions and RV function, applied to a specific clinical situation, which is ARDS. Indeed, pulmonary circulation is always injured in ARDS, and pulmonary hypertension is inherent to the syndrome. Then RV function is especially altered according to the severity of the lung injury and also to the respiratory strategy and the ventilatory settings. Using a systematic approach based on the daily use of echocardiography (transthoracic or transesophageal, which has been reported to be more accurate in this situation) during the first days following mechanical ventilation, intensivists may propose an original strategy in order to prevent or correct RV failure and avoid hemodynamic compromise. Most of the echo parameters with their required relative views were described in the already two cited chapters.

In a large series of more than 700 moderate to severe ARDS ventilated with a lung-protective approach, there has

A. Vieillard-Baron (✉)
Surgical and Medical ICU, University Hospital Ambroise Paré, APHP, Boulogne-Billancourt, France
e-mail: antoine.vieillard-baron@aphp.fr

© Springer Nature Switzerland AG 2020   187
M. Slama (ed.), *Echocardiography in ICU*,
https://doi.org/10.1007/978-3-030-32219-9_20

been reported an incidence of RV failure, named acute cor pulmonale (ACP), of 22% during the first 2 days (Box 20.1 and Figs. 20.1 and 20.2).

Box 20.1 Acute Cor Pulmonale (ACP)

Acute cor pulmonale associates:
- RV dilation.
- Paradoxical septal motion (D-shape).
- Pulmonary hypertension.
- Small left ventricle.
- Impairment of left ventricular filling.

A risk score (1 to 4) for acute cor pulmonale in ARDS patients has also been proposed based on the four factors associated:
- Pneumonia as the cause of ARDS.
- PaO_2/FiO_2 <150 mmHg.
- $PaCO_2$ ≥48 mmHg.
- Driving pressure ≥18 cmH_2O.

The incidence of ACP was:
- Lower than 10% when the score is 0 or 1.
- Around 20% for a score of 2.
- Higher than 30% and 70% for a score of 3 and 4, respectively.

Plateau pressure is a key actor for the development of RV failure, the safety plateau pressure for the right ventricle being below 27 cmH_2O.

An increase in PEEP may lead to significant hypercapnia and RV failure.

In the most severe patients with the lowest lung compliance, increasing the PEEP frequently requires more decrease of the tidal volume to maintain the plateau

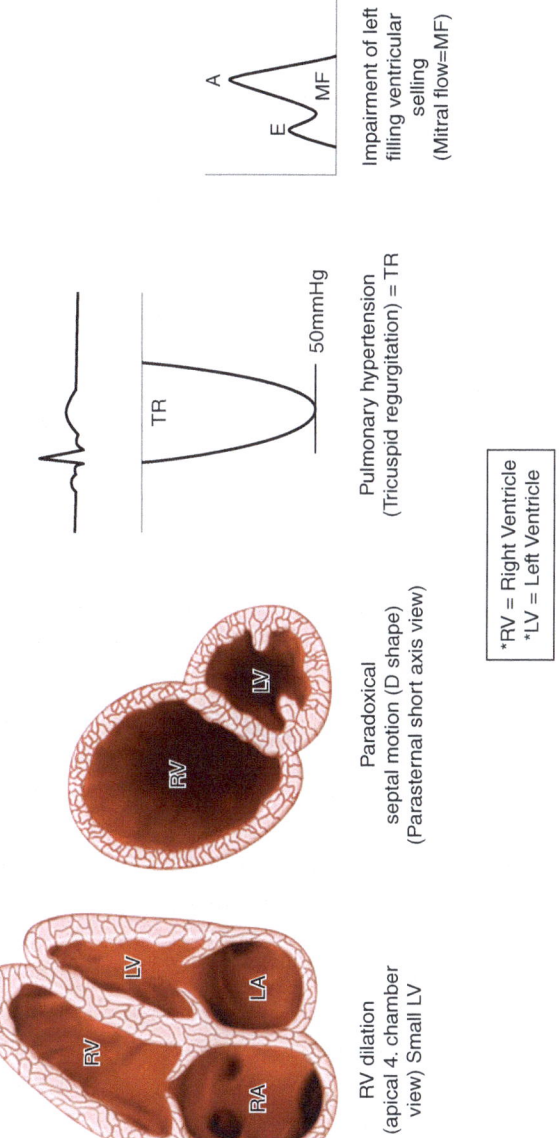

FIGURE 20.1 Acute cor pulmonale

RV dilation
(apical 4. chamber
view) Small LV

Paradoxical
septal motion (D shape)
(Parasternal short axis view)

Pulmonary hypertension
(Tricuspid regurgitation) = TR

Impairment of left
filling ventricular
selling
(Mitral flow=MF)

50mmHg

TR

A

E

MF

*RV = Right Ventricle
*LV = Left Ventricle

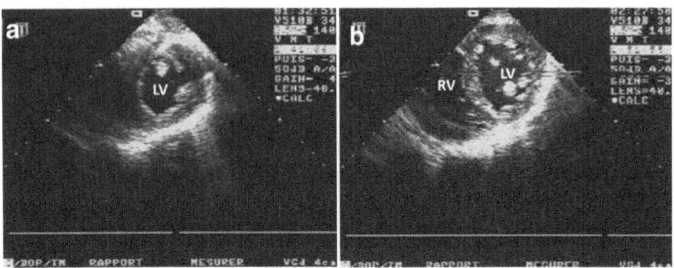

FIGURE 20.2 Deleterious effect of hypercapnia on RV function. Panel a: moderate $PaCO_2$ (52 mmHg). Panel b: severe $PaCO_2$ (72 mmHg) with the same plateau pressure, a lower driving pressure (lower tidal volume), and a higher PEEP (14 versus 7 cmH_2O). Heated and moisture exchanger was removed between panels a and b and replaced by a heated humidifier. *RV* right ventricle, *LV* left ventricle

pressure in the safety limit. Despite a decrease in the instrumental dead space (removal of heat and moisture exchanger for a heated humidifier), $PaCO_2$ may increase very significantly, inducing vasoconstriction of the pulmonary circulation and increased RV afterload. Increase respiratory rate has been reported not to be the panacea for limiting $PaCO_2$ because of its effect on dynamic hyperinflation and intrinsic PEEP. How extracorporeal CO_2 removal will be efficient in patients to control hypercapnia and limit its deleterious effect on the right ventricle has to be evaluated in the future; experimental studies strongly suggest such an effect (Fig. 20.3).

High plateau and driving pressures could be not tolerated by the right ventricle despite a limited tidal volume.

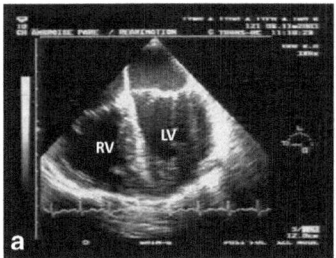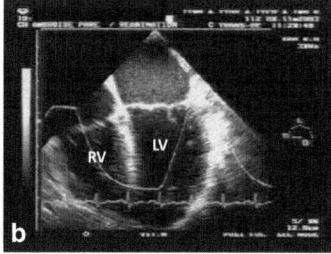

FIGURE 20.3 Plateau and driving pressures too elevated for the right ventricle. Panel a: the plateau pressure was 33 cmH$_2$O, and the driving pressure 28 cmH$_2$O. PaCO$_2$ was 67 mmHg. The patient exhibited severe cor pulmonale. Panel b: plateau pressure and driving pressure were decreased at 26 and 21 cmH$_2$O, respectively, without change in PaCO$_2$. RV appeared less dilated, and hemodynamics was better (increased blood pressure, decreased heart rate)

In this situation, decreasing a little bit more the tidal volume may be beneficial, provided that the instrumental dead space is decreased and the respiratory rate is slightly increased to limit the augmentation of PaCO$_2$. The decrease in such pressures limits the collapse of the pulmonary capillaries by the distending alveoli (West zone 1 or 2).

Prone position, by correcting all the risk factors for RV failure without increasing the PEEP, improves RV function (Fig. 20.4). If and how its beneficial effects on prognosis and on RV function are linked might be evaluated in the future.

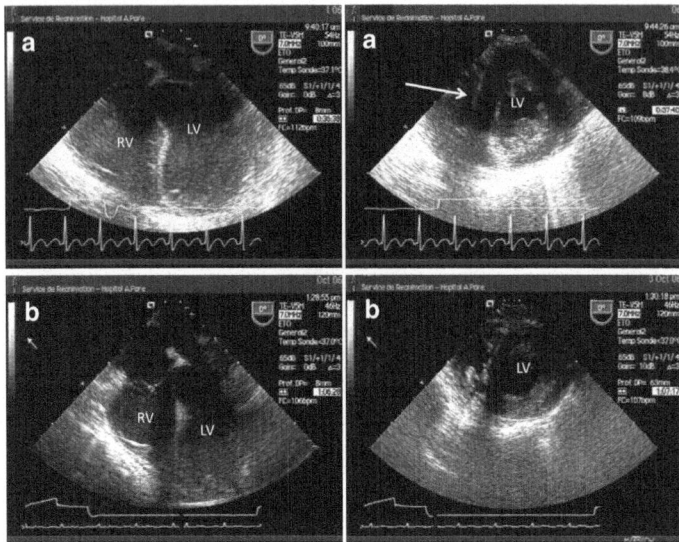

FIGURE 20.4 Effect of the first 18 h of proning in a severe ARDS with a PaO_2/FiO_2 below 100 mmHg. Before the proning session (panel a), the mid-esophageal view (four cavities) showed a major RV dilatation (the right ventricle looks bigger than the left ventricle) and the short-axis transgastric view a paradoxical septal motion (arrow). After the proning (panel b), same views showed normalization of the RV size, as well as of the movement of the interventricular septum. *RV* right ventricle, *LV* left ventricle

Multiple Choice Questions

1. Among the following parameters, which ones have been strictly proven to be at risk of RV failure?

    A. Hyperoxia.
    B. Hypocapnia.
    C. High PEEP.
    D. High plateau pressure (>26 cmH$_2$O).
    E. Hypercapnia.
    Answers: D, E

2. What has been proven (clinically or experimentally) to control the deleterious effect of hypercapnia on RV function?

   A. VA ECMO.
   B. VV ECMO.
   C. High respiratory rate.
   D. Prone position.
   E. Extracorporeal CO_2 removal ($ECCO_2R$).
   Answers: A, D, E

3. A right ventricular protective approach would:

   A. Systematically apply a high PEEP.
   B. Limit the driving pressure.
   C. Decrease the FiO_2.
   D. Largely use proning.
   E. Limit the level of hypercapnia.
   Answers: B, D, E

Suggested Readings

Jardin F, Vieillard-Baron A. Is there a safe plateau pressure in ARDS? The right heart only knows. Intensive Care Med. 2007;33:444–7.

Mekontso-Dessap A, Boissier F, Charron C, et al. Acute cor pulmonale during protective ventilation for acute respiratory distress syndrome: prevalence, predictors, and clinical impact. Intensive Care Med. 2016;42:862–70.

Paternot A, Repessé X, Vieillard-Baron A. Rationale and description of right ventricle-protective ventilation in ARDS. Respir Care. 2016;61:1391–6.

Price L, McAuley D, Marino P, Finney S, Griffiths M, Wort S. Pathophysiology of pulmonary hypertension in acute lung injury. Am J Physiol Lung Cell Mol Physiol. 2012;302(9):L803–15.

Vieillard-Baron A, Charron C, Caille V, et al. Prone position unloads the right ventricle in severe ARDS. Chest. 2007;132:1440–6.

Chapter 21
Pulmonary Embolism

Julien Maizel

21.1 Echocardiography in the Diagnostic Strategy of PE

In the absence of hypotension or shock, the diagnostic algorithm for patients with suspected PE relies on D-dimer and CT angiography but not on echocardiography.

In the presence of hypotension or shock, if CT angiography cannot be performed immediately or if the patient is too unstable, echocardiography should be performed straightway to look for RV dysfunction (Boxes 21.1 and 21.2).

Electronic Supplementary Material The online version of this chapter (https://doi.org/10.1007/978-3-030-32219-9_21) contains supplementary material, which is available to authorized users.

J. Maizel (✉)
Medical ICU, Amiens University Hospital, Amiens, France
e-mail: Maizel.julien@chu-amiens.fr

© Springer Nature Switzerland AG 2020
M. Slama (ed.), *Echocardiography in ICU*,
https://doi.org/10.1007/978-3-030-32219-9_21

Box 21.1 Echocardiographic Signs of Pulmonary Embolism (PE)

Echocardiographic signs associated with acute PE in the context of clinical suspicion

- Visualization of mobile thrombi in the RV and/or emboli in the pulmonary artery (TOE) and/or deep vein thrombosis.
- RV dysfunction: dilatation of the RV.

    - Apical four chambers: RVDA/LVDA >0.6 and paradoxical septum motion.
    - Left parasternal short axis: D-shape and paradoxical septum (Fig. 21.1 and Video 21.1).

- McConnell's sign.

    - Occurs every time acute pulmonary resistances increase, mainly in case of pulmonary embolism but not only.
    - Association of RV dilatation with akinesia of the mid RV free wall and hypercontractility of the RV apex.

- 60 to 60 sign

    - SPAP <60 mmHg.
    - Acceleration time of pulmonary artery <60 ms (Fig. 21.2).

Box 21.2 Risk Assessment Using Echocardiography and Doppler in Pulmonary Embolism (PE)

RV right ventricle, *LV* left ventricle, *SPAP* systolic pulmonary artery pressure, *TAPSE* tricuspid annular plane systolic excursion

Echocardiography in the Prognostic Assessment of PE

- Increased RV/LV end-diastolic area or diameters (>0.6).
- Hypokinesia of the free RV wall.
- Increased SPAP.
- Decreased TAPSE (<12 cm/s).
- Patent foramen ovale.

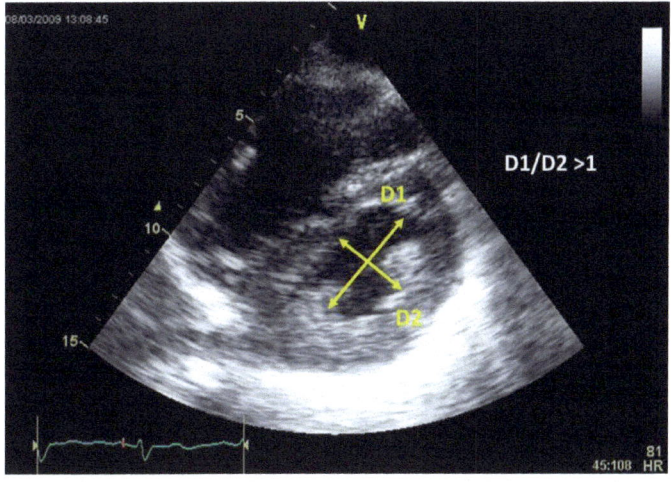

FIGURE 21.1 D-shape. Measurement of the eccentricity index (D1/D2). Normal value ≤1 and in ACP >1

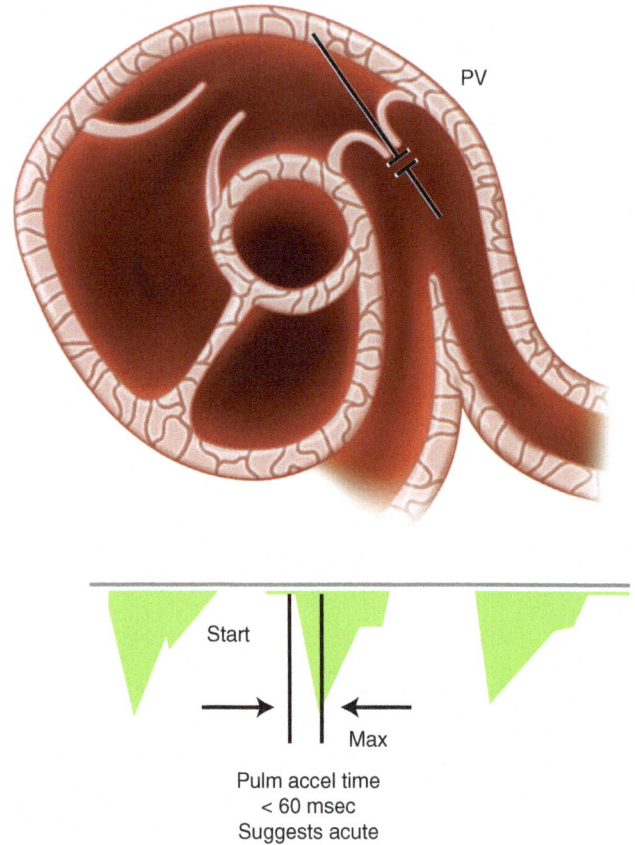

PV

Start

Max

Pulm accel time
< 60 msec
Suggests acute

FIGURE 21.2 Pulmonary flow acceleration time measurement

Multiple Choice Questions

1. Which signs on echocardiography are usually associated with pulmonary embolism?

    A. Paradoxical septal motion.
    B. Left ventricular systolic dysfunction.

C. Hypercontractility of the right ventricle apex.
D. SPAP >60 mmHg.
E. Right ventricle dilatation.
Answers: A, C, E

2. Which signs on echocardiography are usually associated with a poor prognostic in case of pulmonary embolism?

A. E/A mitral flow higher than 3.
B. Right atrial dilatation.
C. Right ventricle systolic dysfunction.
D. Visualization of mobile thrombi in the RV and/or emboli in the pulmonary artery.

Answer: C

Suggested Readings

Konstantinides SV, Torbicki A, Agnelli G, Danchin N, Fitzmaurice D, Galiè N, Gibbs JS, Huisman MV, Humbert M, Kucher N, Lang I, Lankeit M, Lekakis J, Maack C, Mayer E, Meneveau N, Perrier A, Pruszczyk P, Rasmussen LH, Schindler TH, Svitil P, Vonk Noordegraaf A, Zamorano JL, Zompatori M, Task Force for the Diagnosis and Management of Acute Pulmonary Embolism of the European Society of Cardiology (ESC). 2014 ESC guidelines on the diagnosis and management of acute pulmonary embolism. Eur Heart J. 2014;35(43):3033–69.

Rudski LG, Lai WW, Afilalo J, Hua L, Handschumacher MD, Chandrasekaran K, Solomon SD, Louie EK, Schiller NB. Guidelines for the echocardiographic assessment of the right heart in adults: a report from the American Society of Echocardiography endorsed by the European Association of Echocardiography, a registered branch of the European Society of Cardiology, and the Canadian Society of Echocardiography. J Am Soc Echocardiogr. 2010;23(7):685–713.

Chapter 22
Valvulopathy Quantification

Sam Orde

Tips
- Ensure accurate Doppler angles (use off-axis imaging if needed).
- If you suspect significant valvular abnormalities, look 'upstream' and 'downstream'.
- Use dimensionless severity index (DSI), particularly in cases of hyperdynamic circulation or low stroke volume states to avoid over/underestimation of severity.
- Evaluate the aortic valve from several windows (e.g. apical five chambers, apical three chambers, suprasternal).

Continuity Equation
- It is used to determine valve area.
- Flow through one area (e.g. LVOT) is equal to flow through another (e.g. aortic valve) *unless* there is loss/gain

Electronic Supplementary Material The online version of this chapter (https://doi.org/10.1007/978-3-030-32219-9_22) contains supplementary material, which is available to authorized users.

S. Orde (✉)
Nepean Hospital, Sydney, NSW, Australia

© Springer Nature Switzerland AG 2020
M. Slama (ed.), *Echocardiography in ICU*,
https://doi.org/10.1007/978-3-030-32219-9_22

of flow somehow (e.g. significant regurgitation in a valve on the same side of the heart, e.g. aortic or mitral regurgitation).

Tip
- Make multiple measures to ensure accuracy.

Aortic valve stenosis (Case 2: moderate aortic stenosis with aortic regurgitation))

Echocardiography method	Potential findings	Evaluation
2D imaging	Thickened (or abnormal, e.g. bicuspid) aortic valve leaflets Left ventricle hypertrophy Left ventricle and atrial dilation Left ventricle dysfunction	Anatomical aortic valve area by planimetry of the aortic valve in short-axis view (transthoracic or TEE)
Colour Doppler	Chaotic and increased flows in aortic root	
Pulsed wave Doppler	Left ventricle diastolic dysfunction Evaluate LVOT VTI and stroke volume	LVOT VTI (for dimensionless severity index [DSI]) Stroke volume (for continuity equation)
Continuous wave Doppler	Raised peak aortic velocity Raised peak and mean pressure gradient	Valve area by continuity equation (Fig. 22.1)

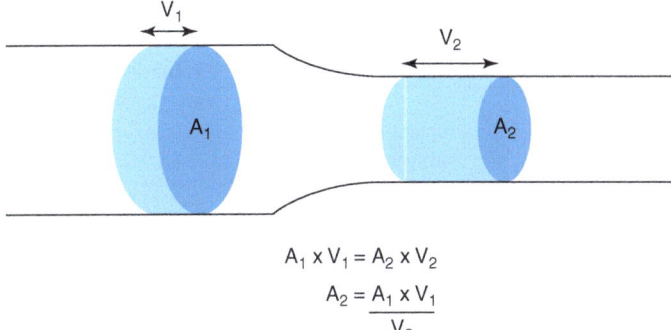

$$A_1 \times V_1 = A_2 \times V_2$$
$$A_2 = \frac{A_1 \times V_1}{V_2}$$

FIGURE 22.1 Continuity Equation

Severity aortic stenosis (Fig. 22.2)

Parameter	Mild	Moderate	Severe
Aortic peak velocity (m/s)	2.6–2.9	3–4	>4
Peak gradient (mmHg)	25–35	36–64	>64
Mean gradient (mmHg)	<20	20–40	>40
Dimensionless severity index	>0.5	0.25–0.5	<0.25
Aortic valve area (cm^2)	>1.5	1–1.5	<1

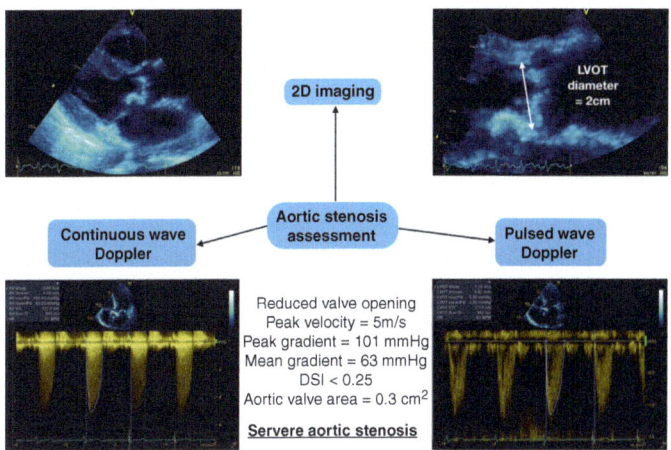

FIGURE 22.2 Aortic valve stenosis assessment

Aortic valve regurgitation

Echocardiography method	Potential findings	Evaluation
2D imaging	Aortic valve structural abnormalities Left ventricle dilation Left ventricle dysfunction Left atrial dilation	Valve leaflets
Colour Doppler	Flow into left ventricle	Aortic regurgitation height vs LVOT diameter Vena contracta
Pulsed wave Doppler	Left ventricle diastolic dysfunction Diastolic mitral regurgitation	Flow reversal in descending aorta
Continuous wave Doppler	Aortic regurgitation flow	Pressure half-time Flow density profile

Severity aortic regurgitation (AR) (Fig. 22.3)

Parameter	Mild	Moderate	Severe
AR jet height vs LVOT diameter (%)	<25%	25–65%	>65%
Vena contracta width (mm)	<3	3–6	>6
Pressure half-time (ms)	>500	200–500	<200
Flow reversal in descending aorta	–	–	+

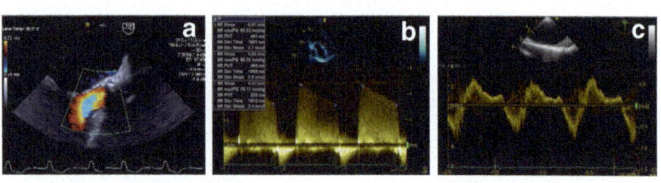

FIGURE 22.3 Aortic valve regurgitation assessment. (**a**) AR jet height vs LVOT diameter. (**b**) Flow reversal in descending aorta. (**c**) Pressure half-time (ms)

Mitral valve stenosis (Case 1: mitral stenosis with mitral regurgitation))

Echocardiography method	Potential findings	Evaluation
2D imaging	Mitral valve leaflet thickening Left atrial dilation	Anatomical mitral valve area by planimetry in short-axis view (transthoracic or TEE)
Colour Doppler	Increased flows into left ventricle	'Candle-flame' appearance in left ventricle
Pulsed wave Doppler	Increased E-wave velocity at mitral valve leaflet tips	Systolic blunting in pulmonary vein flow
Continuous wave Doppler	Decreased slope of E wave in mitral inflow	Transmitral mean pressure gradient Pressure half-time (220/ $T_{1/2}$) Mitral valve area estimation (by continuity equation) Pulmonary hypertension

Severity mitral stenosis (Fig. 22.4)

Parameter	Mild	Moderate	Severe
Mean pressure gradient (mmHg)	<5	5–10	>10
Valve area (cm^2)	>1.5	1–1.5	<1
Systolic pulmonary artery pressures (mmHg)	<30	30–50	>50

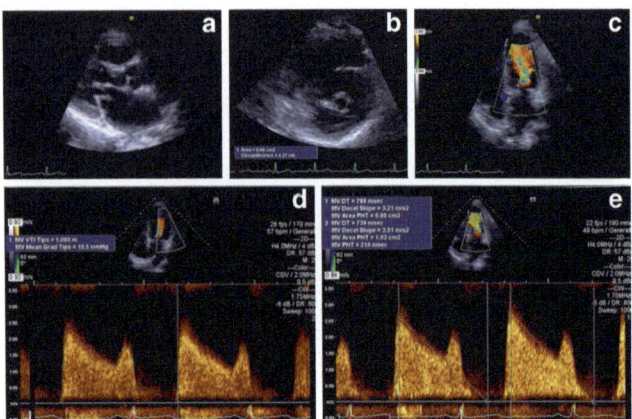

FIGURE 22.4 Mitral stenosis assessment. (**a**) Mitral valve thickening.
(**b**) Mitral valve planimetry. (**c**) Mitral valve inflow on colour
Doppler. (**d**) Mean pressure gradient. (**e**) Pressure half-time (estimating valve area)

Mitral valve regurgitation (Table 22.1, Fig. 22.5)

Echocardiography method	**Potential findings**	**Evaluation**
2D imaging	Mitral valve apparatus abnormalities Mitral annular calcification Left atrial dilation Left ventricle dilation	Mitral annulus dilation Interatrial septum bowed to right
Colour Doppler	Regurgitant flow into left atrium	Regurgitant flow area vs left atrium[a] Vena contracta
Pulsed wave Doppler	Increased E-wave velocity (>1.2 m/s) Systolic pulmonary venous inflow blunting or reversal	Mitral valve VTI/LVOT VTI (NB: as long as no significant aortic regurgitation)
Continuous wave Doppler	Mitral regurgitation jet Pulmonary hypertension	Jet density and symmetry Tricuspid regurgitation

[a]NB: Watch for eccentric jets where the colour Doppler area may under-
estimate the severity of mitral regurgitation (due to Coanda effect)

TABLE 22.1 Factors that increase or reduce the color Doppler jet area

Increases jet area	Reduces jet area
Higher momentum	Lower momentum
Larger regurgitant orifice area	Smaller regurgitant orifice area
Higher velocity (greater pressure gradient)	Lower velocity (lower pressure gradient)
Higher entrainment of flow	Chamber constraint/wall-impinging jet
Lower Nyquist limit	Higher Nyquist limit
Higher Doppler gain	Lower Doppler gain
Far-field beam widening	Far-field attenuation/attenuation by an interposed ultrasound-reflecting structure
Slit-like regurgitant orifice, imaged along the thin, long shape of the orifice	
Multiple orifices	

Severity mitral regurgitation

Parameter	Mild	Moderate	Severe
Jet area (cm^2)	<4	4–8	>8
Jet area: left atrial area (%)	<20	20–40	>40
Vena contracta (mm)	3	3–7	7
Mitral valve VTI: LVOT VTI	–	–	>1
Estimated orifice area (cm^2)	<0.2	0.2–0.4	>0.4

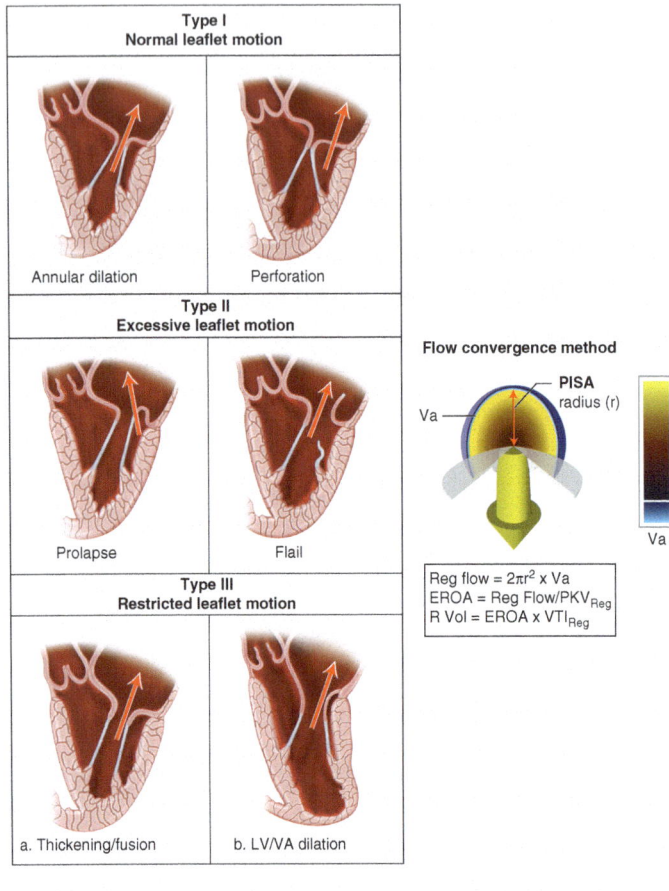

Type I
Normal leaflet motion

Annular dilation   Perforation

Type II
Excessive leaflet motion

Prolapse   Flail

Type III
Restricted leaflet motion

a. Thickening/fusion   b. LV/VA dilation

Flow convergence method

PISA
radius (r)

Va

Va

Reg flow = $2\pi r^2$ x Va
EROA = Reg Flow/PKV_{Reg}
R Vol = EROA x VTI_{Reg}

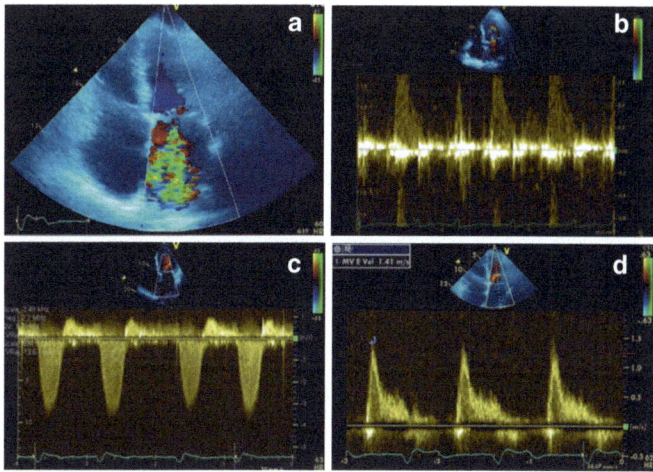

FIGURE 22.5 Mitral regurgitation assessment. (**a**) Colour Doppler. (**b**) Pulmonary venous flow. (**c**) Continuous wave Doppler. (**d**) Mitral valve E-wave velocity

Tricuspid valve regurgitation

Echocardiography method	Potential findings	Evaluation
2D imaging	Tricuspid annular dilation Right ventricle dilation Right atrial dilation	Tricuspid valve abnormalities
Colour Doppler	Tricuspid regurgitation Hepatic vein flow towards probe during systole	Regurgitant jet area Vena contracta
Pulsed wave Doppler	Hepatic vein flow	Hepatic vein systolic flow reversal
Continuous wave Doppler	Tricuspid regurgitation flow	Density of regurgitation flow Assymetrical shape Systolic pulmonary artery pressures ($4 \times TR_{Vmax}$)

Severity tricuspid regurgitation (Fig. 22.6)

Parameter	Mild	Moderate	Severe
Regurgitant jet area	Small Central	Intermediate	Large central jet
Vena contracta (mm)	Not defined	<7	>7
Tricuspid regurgitation continuous Doppler jet	Faint	Filled Parabolic	Dense Assymetrical
Hepatic vein flow	Systolic dominance	Systolic blunting	Systolic flow reversal

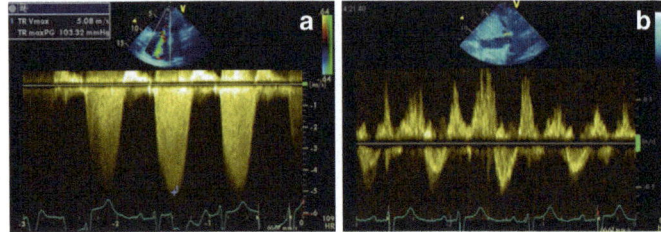

FIGURE 22.6 Tricuspid regurgitation assessment. (**a**) Tricuspid regurgitation continuous wave Doppler trace. (**b**) Hepatic vein flow (systolic flow reversal)

Multiple Choice Questions

1. Which of the following indicates severe mitral regurgitation?

   A. Left atrial dilation.
   B. Interatrial septum bowing to the left.
   C. Left ventricle dilation.
   D. Systolic flow reversal in pulmonary veins.
   E. Dense mitral regurgitation jet.
   Answer: D

2. Which of the following indicates severe aortic regurgitation?

   A. Left ventricle hypertrophy.
   B. Diastolic flow reversal in ascending aorta.
   C. Decreased left ventricle size.
   D. Mitral valve E-wave velocity >1.2 m/s.
   E. Vena contracta 3 mm.
   Answer: B

3. Which of the following indicates severe tricuspid regurgitation?

   A. Right ventricle free wall hypertrophy.
   B. Tricuspid regurgitation Vmax 4 m/s.
   C. Right atrial dilation.
   D. Interventricle septum bowed to left.
   E. Systolic flow reversal in hepatic vein.
   Answer: E

4. Which of the following is FALSE in regard to assessing aortic valve stenosis?

    A. Use B-mode, colour Doppler, pulsed wave and continuous wave Doppler.
    B. Assess with a single view rather than from multiple windows.
    C. Aortic valve stenosis is associated with left ventricle diastolic dysfunction.
    D. Look for left ventricle hypertrophy.
    E. Dimensionless severity index can be very useful, especially in low flow states.

    Answer: B

5. Regarding the continuity equation:

    A. It is used to assess valve area.
    B. It is accurate when there is a cardiac shunt present.
    C. It is used to estimate cardiac output.
    D. It assumes that there are reduced velocities when blood flows through a narrow orifice.
    E. Using the right ventricle outflow tract is more accurate than using the left.

    Answer: A

Chapter 23
Infective Endocarditis

Julien Maizel

Box 23.1 Indications of TOE in Case of Endocarditis Suspicion

Indications of TOE in case of endocarditis suspicion:
- Transoesophageal echocardiography (TOE) must be performed in case of negative.

  – TTE whenever clinical suspicion persists and particularly in case of suboptimal TTE quality.

- TOE should be performed systematically in case of suspicion of endocarditis with prosthetic valve or intracardiac device.

Electronic Supplementary Material   The online version of this chapter (https://doi.org/10.1007/978-3-030-32219-9_23) contains supplementary material, which is available to authorized users.

J. Maizel (✉)
Medical ICU, Amiens University Hospital, Amiens, France
e-mail: Maizel.julien@chu-amiens.fr

- TOE is also systematically indicated in patients with positive TTE to look for local complications (except for isolated right-sided native valve infective endocarditis with good-quality TTE).

Box 23.2 Endocarditis Lesions (Figs. 23.1 and 23.2)

Echocardiogram lesions positive for IE:

- Vegetation: oscillating or nonoscillating intracardiac mass on valve or other endocardial structures or on implanted intracardiac material.
- Abscess: necrosis and purulent material not communicating with the cardiovascular lumen; perivalvular area with abnormal echodensity (hyper- or hypo-) appearance usually thickened and/or non-homogeneous.
- Pseudoaneurysm: perivalvular circulating neocavity communicating with the cardiovascular lumen; perivalvular anechoic space, with color flow circulation.
- Perforation: dehiscence in the endocardial valvular tissue traversed by colour Doppler flow activity.
- Fistula: communication through a perforation between two cavities detected by colour Doppler flow.

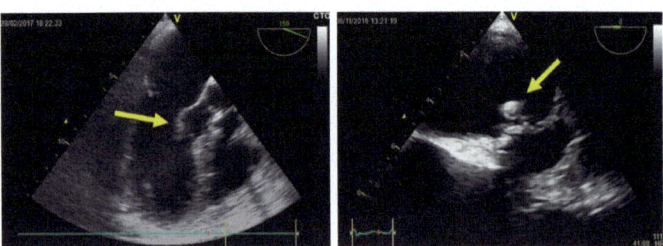

FIGURE 23.1 Vegetation on mitral valve (TEE examination)

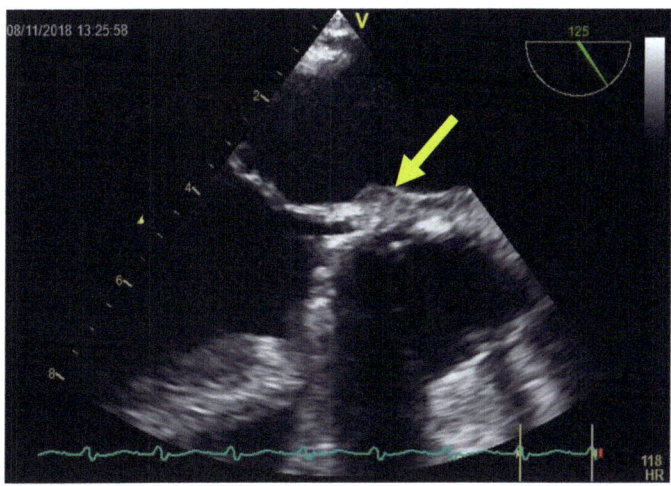

FIGURE 23.2 Abscess on mitral annulus

- Valve aneurysm: saccular bulging of valvular tissue on bi-dimensional.
- New dehiscence of a prosthetic valve.
- New para-valvular regurgitation with or without rocking motion of the prosthesis.

Box 23.3 Differential Diagnosis of Infective Vegetation

Differential diagnosis of infective vegetation:
- Thrombi.
- Chordal rupture.
- Valve fibroelastoma.
- Myxomatous valve disease.
- Strands.
- Libman-Sacks lesions (lupus).
- Marantic vegetation.

Box 23.4 Echocardiographic Findings of Poor Outcome
(Fig. 23.3)

Echocardiographic findings of poor outcome:
- Periannular complications.
- Severe left-sided valve regurgitation.
- Low left ventricular ejection fraction.
- Pulmonary hypertension.
- Large vegetation (>10 mm).
- Severe prosthetic valve dysfunction.
- Premature mitral valve closure and other signs of elevated diastolic pressures.

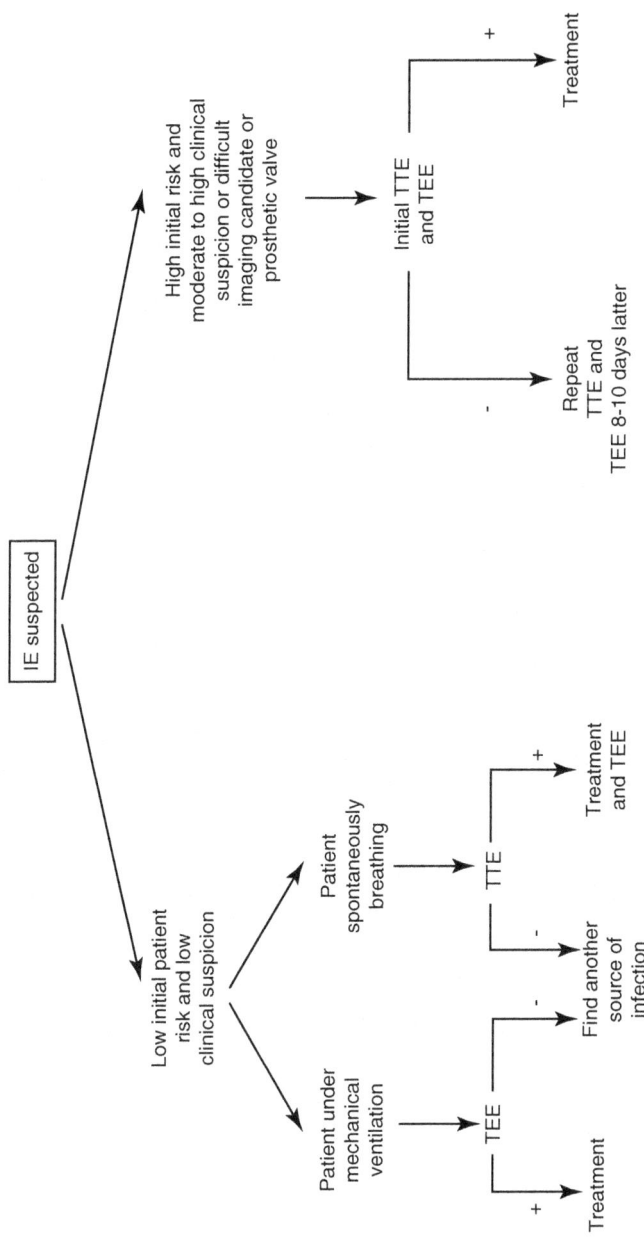

FIGURE 23.3 Algorithm in case of suspicion of infective endocarditis (EI)

Suggested Readings

Afonso L, Kottam A, Reddy V, Penumetcha A. Echocardiography in infective endocarditis: state of the art. Curr Cardiol Rep. 2017;19:127.

Bai AD, Steinberg M, Showler A, Burry L, Bhatia RS, Tomlinson GA, Bell CM, Morris AM. Diagnostic accuracy of transthoracic echocardiography for infective endocarditis findings using transesophageal echocardiography as the reference standard: a meta-analysis. J Am Soc Echocardiogr. 2017;30:639–46.

Chapter 24
Prosthetic Valve Evaluation

Stephen J. Huang

24.1 Types of Prosthetic Heart Valves

There are two main types of prosthetic heart valves (PHV): mechanical and biological (Fig. 24.1) [1, 2]. The use of biological prosthesis has been increasing over the last 15–20 years despite mechanical prosthesis offering better long-term survival benefits [3].

24.2 Common Prosthetic Valve Complications

Common PHV complications include thromboembolic and haemorrhagic events, endocarditis, nonstructural dysfunction (such as perivalvular leaks and pannus ingrowth), and prosthesis-patient mismatch (PPM) [4].

S. J. Huang (✉)
Intensive Care Unit, Nepean Hospital, University of Sydney
Nepean Clinical School, Sydney, NSW, Australia
e-mail: Stephen.huang@sydney.edu.au

© Springer Nature Switzerland AG 2020
M. Slama (ed.), *Echocardiography in ICU*,
https://doi.org/10.1007/978-3-030-32219-9_24

219

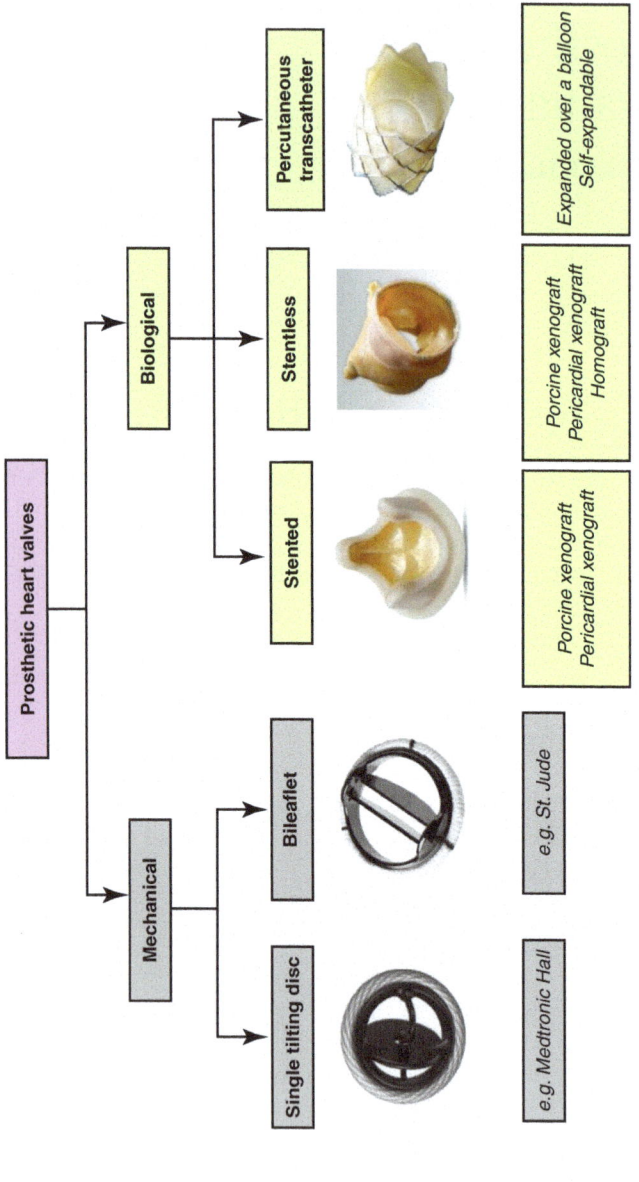

FIGURE 24.1 Common types of prosthetic valves. Mechanical prosthetic heart valves also include "caged ball" valve, which is now discontinued

Patients with PHV are at higher risk of thromboembolic events, and the risk is higher with mechanical valve and with mitral prosthesis. Concomitant risk factors such as atrial fibrillation and left atrial dilatation, poor ventricular function, and history of thromboembolism further increase the risk. These patients are also at higher risk of endocarditis due to tissue degeneration in bioprosthetic valve over time or to a lack of endothelialization in the mechanical valve surface in the early stage. In the long term, the risk of endocarditis is similar between the two types of valves [5].

PPM refers to situations where the effective orifice area (EOA) is too small, resulting in the cardiac output not being able to meet the body's demand. Common causes are when the prosthesis is too small in relation to the body size or there is obstruction in the prosthesis. PPM therefore poses a hemodynamic risk to patients with shock. The impact of PPM is most significant in patients with poor LV function. Mitral PPM may also result in pulmonary hypertension.

24.3   Echocardiographic Evaluation of Prosthetic Valve

Echocardiographic evaluation of prosthetic valve in ICU can be summarized as follows:

- 2D evaluation of the prosthetic valve.
- 2D evaluation of cardiac chamber size and function.
- Color Doppler examination of regurgitation.
- Continuous-wave (CW) and pulsed-wave (PW) Doppler evaluation of pathologic obstruction, pathologic regurgitation, and patient-prosthesis mismatch (Fig. 24.2).

Evaluation of prosthetic valve using transthoracic echocardiography is possible but is limited, especially in the prosthetic mitral valve.

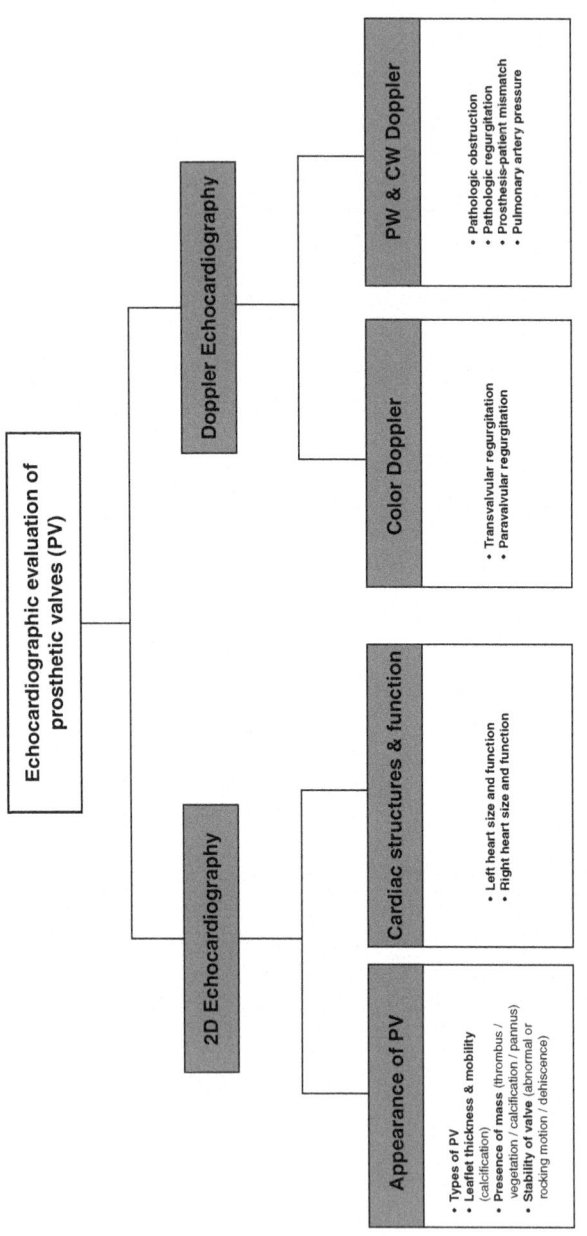

FIGURE 24.2 Echocadiographic evaluation of prosthetic valves

24.4   Information Required for Full Echocardiographic Evaluation

Wherever possible, the following information is helpful and should be collected in the evaluation of prosthetic valve in an intensive care patient:

- Clinical information.
- Type and size of prosthesis.
- Height and weight (body surface area).
- Hemodynamic status, such as blood pressure and heart rate.
- Baseline study, if available.

24.5   Evaluation Algorithm

24.5.1   PPM vs. Prosthetic Dysfunction

Evaluation starts off by measuring the transvalvular mean pressure gradient (Fig. 24.3). A high mean pressure gradient suggests high-flow state, PPM, or prosthetic dysfunction. High-flow state can be identified by a normal Doppler velocity index (DVI), defined as:

$$DVI = \frac{VTI_{LVOT}}{VTI_{PV}}$$

where VTI_{LVOT} and VTI_{PV} are the velocity time integrals of LV outflow tract (LVOT) and the prosthetic valve (PV) (Fig. 24.4). LVOT Doppler signals are obtained from flow acceleration in the prosthetic aortic valve, approximately 0.5–1.0 cm below the sewing ring (LV side). As assessment of the left heart prosthetic valve relies on accurate LVOT Doppler assessment, care must be taken to minimize LVOT velocity measurement error, especially Doppler angle error (see Chap. 1).

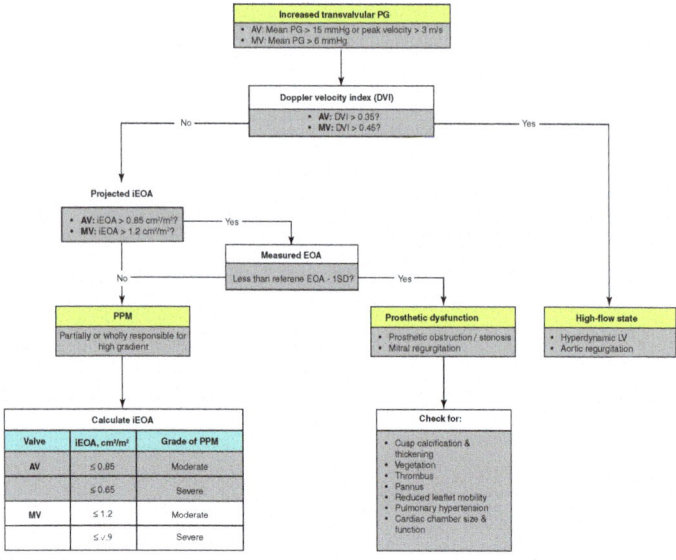

Figure 24.3 Assessment algorithm for prosthetic valve. Projected iEOA is the indexed EOA calculated using the manufacturer-provided EOA for the type and size of prosthetic valve. Manufacturer-provided EOA values can be found in various sources (e.g., ref.2). *AV* aortic valve, *DVI* Doppler velocity index, *EOA* effective orifice area, *iEOA* indexed EOA, *MV* mitral valve, *PG* pressure gradient, *PPM* prosthesis-patient mismatch

A normal EOA, calculated using continuity equation (see Chap. 22), suggests prosthetic dysfunction, whereas abnormal EOA suggests PPM when DVI is reduced (Fig. 24.3).

24.5.2   Regurgitations

A small leakage (regurgitation) is necessary in PV to prevent blood stasis and thrombus formation. This is known as washing effect. This leakage is characterized by short duration, narrow, and symmetrical regurgitation jets. Significant

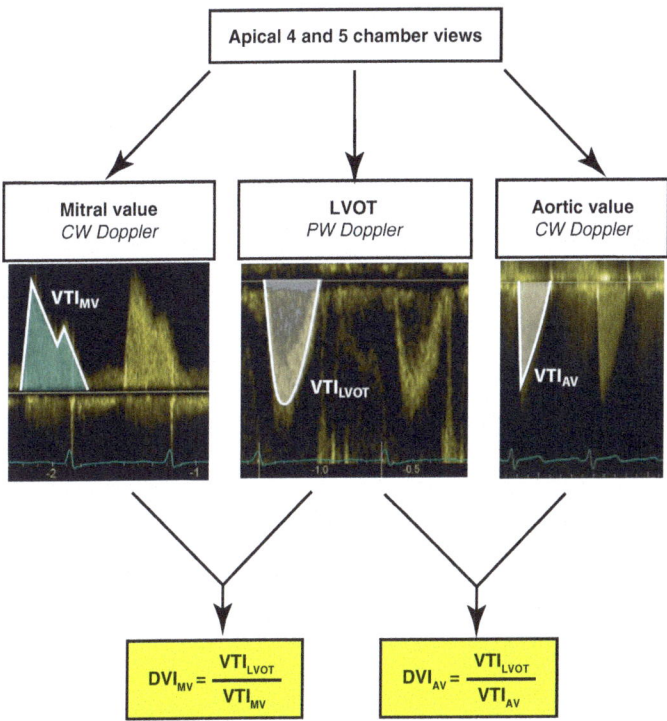

FIGURE 24.4 Calculation of DVI

regurgitation can be transvalvular or paravalvular. Transvalvular jets can be caused by a flail bioprosthetic cusp or the presence of pannus or the thrombus interfering with a leaflet closure. Paravalvular jets are caused by dehiscence. The location and size of the paravalvular jet should be recorded. For aortic prostheses, the extent of paravalvular regurgitation can be reported as a percentage of circumference. For mitral prostheses, severity of regurgitation can be reported as regurgitant volume or fraction [6] (Table 24.1 and Fig. 24.5).

TABLE 24.1 Severity of aortic and mitral valve prosthesis regurgitations

	Mild	**Moderate**	**Severe**
Aortic and mitral prostheses			
Regurgitant volume (ml)	<30	30–59	≥60
Regurgitant fraction (%)	<30	30–49	≥50
Paravalvular aortic regurgitation:			
% circumference	<10	10–20	>20

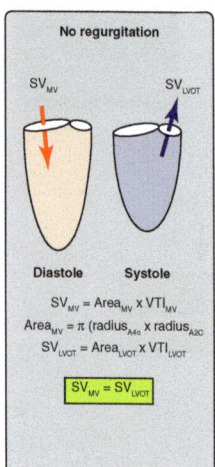 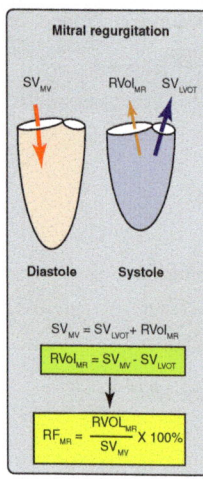 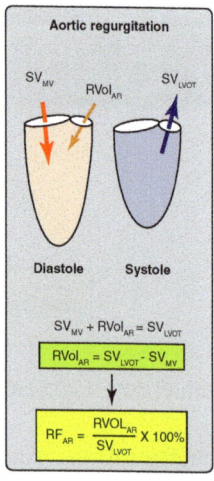

FIGURE 24.5 Calculation of regurgitant volume and fraction. Based on the principle of conservation of mass, blood volume (stroke volume (SV)) entering the LV through mitral valve (MV) is the same as the volume exiting the LV through LVOT provided there is no regurgitation (continuity equation principle). SV is calculated by multiplying the area of the valve by the VTI. Note that the area of MV is the product of π and the radii obtained at apical four chambers (A4C) and apical two chambers (A2C). Where either mitral (MR) or aortic (AR) regurgitation is present, the regurgitant volume (RVol) will need to be taken into account to ensure that the total volume entering is the same as exiting the LV. Regurgitant fraction (RF) is the ratio of RVol to SV of the same valve. Note that when both aortic and mitral regurgitations are present, RVol and RF cannot be calculated using this method

Multiple Choice Questions

1. Prosthesis-patient mismatch refers to:

   A. Rejection of the valve by the body
   B. A large-size valve being transplanted to a small patient
   C. Size of the valve unable to meet the demand of the cardiac output
   D. Material of the valve not suitable to the patient
   Answer: C

2. Which of the following is false?

   A. Assessing pulmonary artery pressure is necessary in prosthetic mitral valve regurgitation
   B. Poor LV function may exacerbate prosthesis-patient mismatch
   C. Any prosthetic valve regurgitations are abnormal
   D. Reduced leaflet mobility in mechanical valve can be caused by vegetation.
   Answer: C

3. Which of the following echocardiographic modality is not necessary for prosthetic valve evaluation in ICU?

   A. 2D imaging (B-mode)
   B. 3D imaging
   C. Color flow Doppler
   D. Pulsed-wave Doppler
   Answer: B

4. Which of the following about DVI is false?

   A. It is a dimensionless parameter
   B. It is the ratio of peak LVOT velocity to peak prosthetic transvalvular velocity
   C. It is useful for grading PPM
   D. DVI is less in significant prosthetic aortic valve regurgitation
   Answer: B

5. Which of the following is less of a challenge in prosthetic valve evaluation?

   A. Shadowing artifact in mechanical mitral prostheses
   B. Ringing down artifact in mechanical mitral prostheses
   C. Visualization of mitral regurgitation in TTE
   D. Visualization of aortic regurgitation in TTE
   Answer: D

6. Which of the following statement is true?

   A. Prosthetic mitral valve EOA can be calculated using pressure half time (PHT), i.e. 220/PHT
   B. Reporting heart rate is important in mitral valve inflow mean pressure gradient
   C. Vena contracta is important in evaluation
   D. A mean pressure gradient or peak velocity that is higher than the native valve should always be a concern
   Answer: B. Heart rate affects diastolic filling and hence will affect the pressure gradient. High heart rate is associated with higher gradient due to insufficient diastolic time to fill up the LV. As a result, the left atrial pressure increases as the preload increases

References

1. Pibarot P, Dumesnil JG. Prosthetic heart valves. Circulation. 2009;119(7):1034–48.
2. Zoghbi WA, Chambers JB, Dumesnil JG, Foster E, Gottdiener JS, Grayburn PA, et al. Recommendations for evaluation of prosthetic valves with echocardiography and doppler ultrasound: a report from the American Society of Echocardiography's guidelines and standards committee and the task force on prosthetic valves, developed in conjunction with the American College of Cardiology Cardiovascular Imaging Committee, Cardiac Imaging Committee of the American Heart Association, the European Association of Echocardiography, a registered branch of the European Society of Cardiology, the Japanese Society of Echocardiography and the Canadian Society of Echocardiography, endorsed by the

American College of Cardiology Foundation, American Heart Association, European Association of Echocardiography, a registered branch of the European Society of Cardiology, the Japanese Society of Echocardiography, and Canadian Society of Echocardiography. J Am Soc Echocardiogr. 2009;22(9):975–1014.

3. Goldstone AB, Chiu P, Baiocchi M, Lingala B, Patrick WL, Fischbein MP, et al. Mechanical or biologic prostheses for aortic-valve and mitral-valve replacement. N Engl J Med. 2017;377(19):1847–57.

4. Misawa Y. Valve-related complications after mechanical heart valve implantation. Surg Today. 2015;45(10):1205–9.

5. Nagpal A, Sohail MR, Steckelberg JM. Prosthetic valve endocarditis: state of the heart. Clin Invest. 2012;2(8):803–17.

6. Pibarot P, Dumesnil JG. Doppler echocardiographic evaluation of prosthetic valve function. Heart. 2011;98(1):69–78.

Chapter 25
Myocardial Infarction and Complications

Sam Orde

Tips:

- Multiple views should be used to assess for regional wall motion abnormalities.
- Parasternal short-axis view is very useful to confirm regional wall motion abnormalities: compare one side with the other and opposite segments.
- Subcostal short-axis views can be useful in difficult to image patients.
- Know myocardial territories supplied by specific coronary arteries. If there are regional wall motion abnormalities outside of these territories, consider stress-induced cardiomyopathies.
- Thinned, increased echogenicity and akinetic segments may indicate chronic ischaemia.
- In areas of akinetic motion, look for potential thrombus (use off-axis imaging if needed).

Electronic Supplementary Material The online version of this chapter (https://doi.org/10.1007/978-3-030-32219-9_25) contains supplementary material, which is available to authorized users.

S. Orde (✉)
Nepean Hospital, Sydney, NSW, Australia

© Springer Nature Switzerland AG 2020
M. Slama (ed.), *Echocardiography in ICU*,
https://doi.org/10.1007/978-3-030-32219-9_25

231

25.1   Regional Wall Motion and Coronary Artery Territories (Table 25.1)

TABLE 25.1 Regional wall motion assessment and scoring (see Fig. 25.1)

Motion	Score	Definition
Normal	1	Increase in systolic thickening >50%
Hypokinesis	2	Increase in systolic thickening <50%
Akinetic	3	Systolic thickening <10%
Dyskinetic	4	Segment is thinned and moves outwards during systole

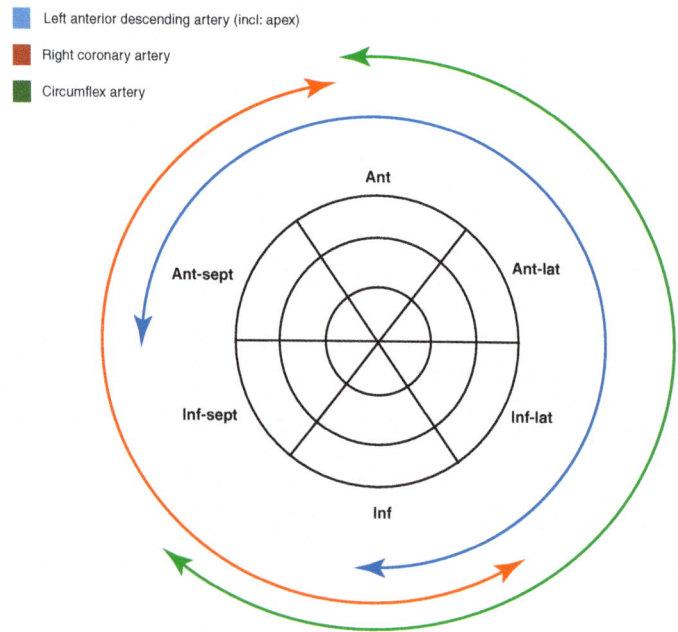

FIGURE 25.1 'Bulls-eye' view of the left ventricle 16-segment regional wall motion (a 17-segment model is also used with an apical 'cap'), as if looking up at the heart from the apex. The outer circle represents the base of the heart, the inner circle the apex

25.2   Complications of Myocardial Ischaemia

(a) **Heart failure and cardiogenic shock** (see *video/case*).

- Assess for regional wall motion abnormalities.
- LV dilation can lead to mitral annular dilation.

(b) **Right ventricle infarction** (see *video/case*).

- Associated with right ventricle failure.
- Right ventricle free wall dysfunction associated with inferior left ventricle basal/mid- ventricle hypo/akinesis.

(c) **Pericardial effusion/pericarditis** (Dressler's syndrome).

- Rarely associated with tamponade.
- Acute response; clinical correlation important.

(d) **Thrombus formation** (in areas of akinesis or aneurysmal segments).

- Associated with areas of low flow (see Fig. 25.2): akinetic or aneurysmal segments, most commonly seen in the apical regions.
- Can be associated with spontaneous echo contrast.

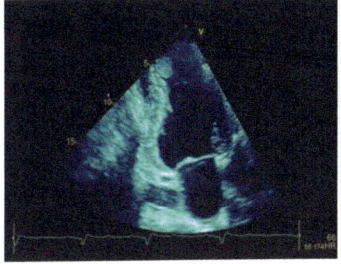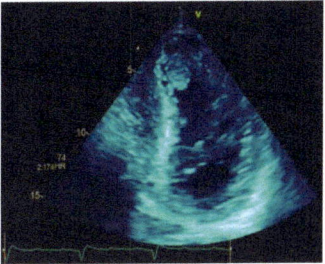

FIGURE 25.2 (+ associated videos) Akinetic and thinned apical left ventricle associated with low flow state. Please note: in standard view thrombus can be missed; hence, there is a need for off-axis imaging

(e) **Ventricle septal rupture** (see Fig. 25.3):

- Acute ventricle septal defect is formed from myocardial rupture as a result of a weakened structure due to ischaemia.
- Off-axis imaging may be required to visualise the defect.
- A turbulent, systolic, high-velocity, left-to-right shunt may be seen (e.g., colour Doppler, as well as continuous wave Doppler).
- It is associated with haemodynamic instability and high mortality.

(f) **Mitral regurgitation from myocardial ischaemia** (see Fig. 25.4).

- Different mechanisms for mitral regurgitation associated with myocardial ischaemia (see Table 25.2).
- May present with symptoms of raised left atrial pressure (shortness of breath, pulmonary oedema).
- Severity of eccentric mitral regurgitation often underestimated by colour Doppler. Review pulmonary veins for systolic flow blunting or reversal of flow indicating significant regurgitation).

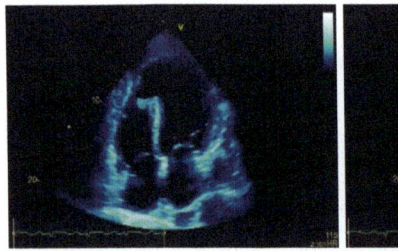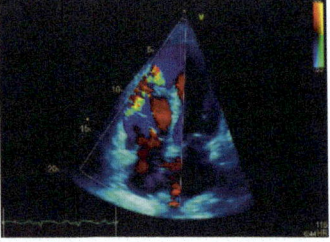

FIGURE 25.3 (+ associated videos) Ventricle septal rupture from acute infarction

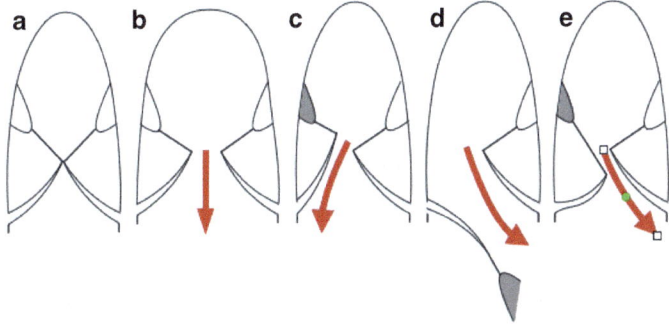

FIGURE 25.4 Mechanisms of mitral regurgitation associated with myocardial ischaemia: (**a**) normal, (**b**) left ventricle annular dilation from heart failure, (**c**) tethering of mitral valve chordae from an underlying ischaemic area, (**d**) papillary muscle rupture (typically posteromedial papillary muscle as sole coronary artery blood supply), (**e**) prolapsed mitral valve from chordae rupture or papillary muscle weakness

TABLE 25.2 Mechanisms of mitral regurgitation associated with myocardial ischaemia

Mechanism of mitral regurgitation	Regurgitation direction	Acute vs. chronic	Figure
Normal	–	–	25.4a
Left ventricle dilation from ischaemia	Central	Chronic	25.4b
Tethering from ischaemic area (inadequate mitral valve coaptation)	Same direction to ischaemic area	Acute or chronic	25.4c
Papillary muscle rupture[a]	Opposite direction to ruptured papillary muscle	Acute	25.4d
Mitral valve prolapse (inadequate papillary muscle contraction)	Opposite direction to ruptured papillary muscle	Acute or chronic	25.4e

[a]Typically associated with inferior infarctions with anteriorly directed jet associated with acute pulmonary oedema, due to posteromedial papillary muscle rupture as only single coronary artery blood supply by the circumflex coronary artery

Multiple Choice Questions

1. Which is the most common complication of myocardial infarction?

    A. Ventricular septal rupture.
    B. Rupture papillary muscle.
    C. Tamponade.
    D. Regional wall motion abnormality.
    Answer: D

2. You are called to see an acutely haemodynamically unstable 70-year-old female 3 days after suffering from STEMI. Angiography found 90% left anterior descending artery stenosis and 100% circumflex artery stenosis. Which of the following is the LEAST likely cause?

    A. Left ventricle dilation.
    B. Ventricle septal rupture.
    C. Mitral valve prolapse.
    D. Posteromedial papillary muscle rupture.
    Answer: A

3. Which of the following is true regarding acute papillary muscle rupture from myocardial infarction?

    A. The anterolateral papillary muscle is most likely affected.
    B. The acute mitral regurgitation flow is in the opposite direction of the affected area of ischaemia.
    C. Right coronary artery occlusion is the most likely culprit coronary artery.
    D. It is a relatively benign complication from a myocardial infarction.
    Answer: B

Chapter 26
Acute Diseases of the Thoracic Aorta

Philippe Vignon

Acute diseases of the thoracic aorta can be divided into two entities encountered in distinct clinical settings: the acute aortic syndrome (AAS), which embraces emergency conditions involving the aorta with similar clinical characteristics, and blunt aortic injuries (BAI) resulting from severe thoracic trauma.

_____

Electronic Supplementary Material   The online version of this chapter (https://doi.org/10.1007/978-3-030-32219-9_26) contains supplementary material, which is available to authorized users.

_____

P. Vignon (✉)
Medical-Surgical Intensive Care Unit, Dupuytren Teaching Hospital, Limoges, France

Inserm CIC-P 1435, Dupuytren Teaching Hospital, Limoges, France
e-mail: philippe.vignon@unilim.fr

© Springer Nature Switzerland AG 2020   237
M. Slama (ed.), _Echocardiography in ICU_,
https://doi.org/10.1007/978-3-030-32219-9_26

Box 26.1: Aortic diseases

AAS results from various acute aortic diseases and is associated with a potential risk of lethal aortic rupture [Fig. 26.1]:

1. Dissection
2. Intramural aortic hematoma
3. Penetrating atherosclerotic aortic ulcer
4. Aneurysm
5. False aneurysm.

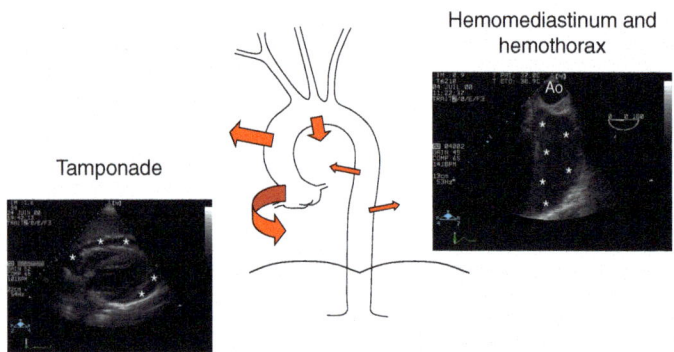

FIGURE 26.1 Acute diseases of the thoracic aorta are life-threatening conditions due to weakened aortic wall and the risk of blood extravasation at various anatomical sites (red arrows). Blood extravasation usually occurs in the region where aortic pressure is the highest (typically the ascending aorta, within the pericardial sac or not) or where the aortic wall is the more severely injured (typically the aortic isthmus for blunt aortic injuries). Echocardiography allows identifying extravasation signs in corresponding normally virtual anatomical spaces: hemopericardium (left panel, asterisks), hemomediastinum, hemothorax (right panel, asterisks)

Box 26.2: Risk factors for AAA

Risk factors for AAS are:

1. Medical history of aortic or Marfan disease
2. Characteristic chest pain (severely intense, tearing, throbbing, and migratory)
3. Presence of hypotension, shock, or perfusion deficit.

BAI occur primarily in the anatomical region of aortic isthmus located between the takeoff of the left subclavian artery and the first intercostal arteries.

The main risk factor for BAI is violent deceleration accidents, which generate high-energy shearing forces acting maximally at the level of the aortic isthmus located between the relatively mobile aortic arch and the tightly fixed descending thoracic aorta.

Transthoracic echocardiography (TTE) is the first-line imaging modality to assess patients with AAS, especially when hemodynamically unstable, whereas transesophageal echocardiography (TEE) constitutes a valuable diagnostic adjunct in ventilated patients sustaining BAI. Both the AAS when involving the ascending aorta (Fig. 26.2) and subadventitial BAI (Fig. 26.3) require emergency correction to avoid lethal rupture. In contrast, AAS involving solely the descending aorta in the absence of complication and superficial BAI can be safely managed conservatively, with a strict control of the blood pressure.

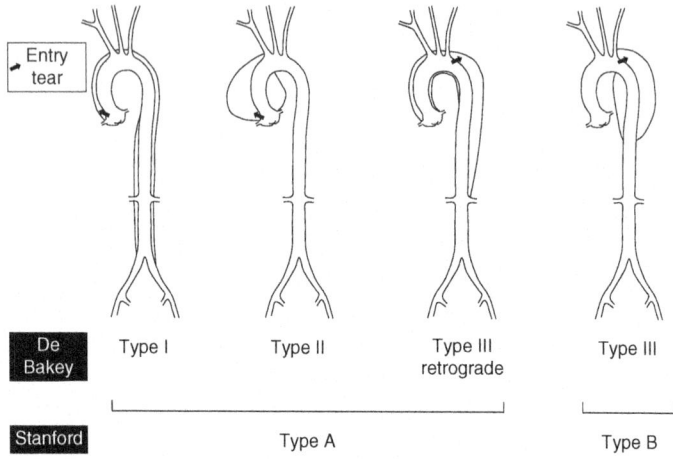

FIGURE 26.2 Schematic representation of different anatomical types of acute aortic dissections according to the De Backey and Stanford classifications. Involvement of the ascending aorta requires prompt surgery

26.1   Acute Aortic Syndrome

Box 26.3: Cardiac complications of acute aortic syndrome

Early cardiac complications of acute aortic syndrome:
- Tamponade (blood extravasation within the pericardium)
- Acute myocardial infarction (extension of dissection to coronary arteries)
- Massive aortic regurgitation (acute dilatation of aortic annulus, intussusception of intimal flap in left ventricular outflow tract, dissected aortic cusps)
- Less frequently, acute circulatory failure resulting from hemorrhagic shock when blood extravasation occurs within a usually virtual internal space (hemomediastinum, hemothorax).

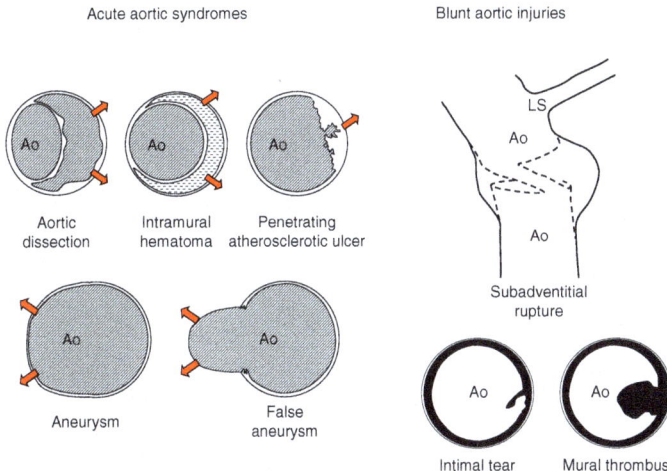

FIGURE 26.3 Schematic illustration of the main acute diseases of the thoracic aorta. Acute aortic syndromes share a common clinical presentation while encompassing various causative conditions that all can lead ultimately to sudden death due to adventitial rupture (red arrows). Among them, acute aortic dissections and intraparietal hematomas are the most frequent. Blunt aortic injuries result from violent deceleration accident and involve primarily the aortic isthmus. When subadventitial, aortic disruption results in a false aneurysm formation (adventitia under pressure), which reflects the threat of lethal rupture. In contrast, intimal tears potentially associated with mural thrombus is too superficial and localized to exert an excessive adventitial pressure; hence, it can be safely managed conservatively. *Ao* aortic lumen, *LS* left subclavian artery

TTE should be performed first since it is rapid to obtain and strictly noninvasive. In a patient with AAS and shock, TTE should seek for a hemopericardium, which reflects underlying blood extravasation and prompts rapid surgery (Fig. 26.1).

The presence of a dilated aortic root associated with a new-onset aortic insufficiency is highly suggestive of AAS involving the ascending aorta.

The absence of intimal flap fails to rule out the diagnosis since TTE lacks sensitivity and AAS may be related to other less prevalent acute aortic diseases than dissection (Fig. 26.3). Intimal flap must be distinguished from intraluminal linear artifacts, which are frequently generated within the ascending aorta by TEE (Video 26.1). In unstable patients who cannot undergo a contrast-enhanced computed tomography, TEE may be advantageously performed during surgery in a stabilized patient under general anesthesia for optimal tolerance and safety (Table 26.1). When compared with initial goal-oriented TTE examination, TEE yields additional information in depicting the underlying acute aortic disease responsible for AAS and potentially associated cardiac complications or extravasation signs (Table 26.1, Figs. 26.4 and 26.5) (Video 26.2).

26.2   Blunt Aortic Injuries

TEE provides accurate visualization of the aortic isthmus, while TTE is not suited for BAI diagnosis (Videos 26.3, 26.4, and 26.5). In addition to clearly distinguish subadventitial

TABLE 26.1   Echocardiographic findings to seek for when assessing a patient with hypotension or shock and suspected acute aortic syndrome

Transthoracic echocardiography	Transesophageal echocardiography
Signs of blood extravasation[a]: • Hemopericardium ± tamponade • Left hemothorax[b]	*Signs of blood extravasation*[a]: • Hemopericardium ± tamponade • Left hemothorax, hemomediastinum[b]

Indirect signs of involvement of the ascending aorta[a]:
• Dilatation (symmetrical) of the ascending aorta
• New-onset aortic insufficiency (color Doppler)
	Indirect signs of involvement of the ascending aorta[a]:
	• Dilatation (symmetrical) of the ascending aorta
	• New-onset aortic insufficiency (color Doppler):
	  Aortic root dilatation
	  Intussusception of the intimal flap
	  Dissected aortic cusp

TABLE 26.1 (continued)

Transthoracic echocardiography	Transesophageal echocardiography
Specific findings:	*Specific findings*:
• Aortic dissection: Intimal flap (mobile) New regional wall motion abnormality[c]	• Aortic dissection: Intimal flap (mobile) Presence of two distinct channels (true channel of smaller size) Low flow velocity ± thrombus in false channel Entry tear ± reentry tear New regional wall motion abnormality[c]
	• Intramural hematoma: Circular or crescent-shaped thickening of the aortic wall >5 mm Absence of detectable blood flow within wall
	• Penetrating atherosclerotic ulcer: Penetrating lesion within a heavily atherosclerotic and calcified aortic wall, Possible association of a localized hematoma or false aneurysm formation

[a]Warning sign requiring emergency surgery
[b]In the presence of hemorrhagic shock secondary to blood extravasation associated with an acute disease of the descending thoracic aorta; right hemothorax is less frequent
[c]Reflecting the extension of dissection to coronary arteries

BAI which require prompt correction from more superficial lesions (Fig. 26.3), TEE allows identification of associated blunt cardiac injuries and helps guiding acute management including endovascular stenting [1–3].

Echocardiographic signs of subadventitial aortic disruption should be distinguished from those associated with aortic dissection (Fig. 26.6), which is rarely due to severe blunt chest trauma (Table 26.2), since they are distinct entities (Fig. 26.7).

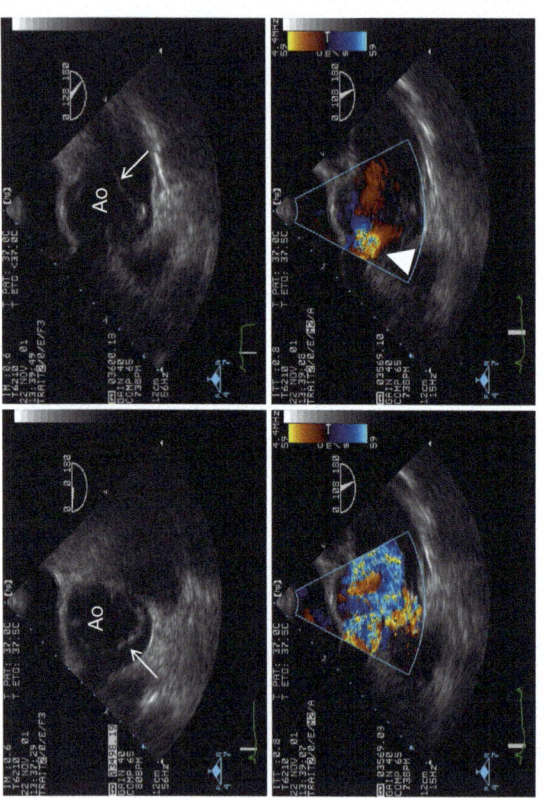

FIGURE 26.4 Acute aortic dissection involving the ascending aorta depicted by transesophageal echocardiography. In both the mid-esophageal transverse (0°, upper left) and longitudinal (120°, upper right) views, two-dimensional imaging depicts an intimal flap within the dilated ascending aorta (arrow). In the longitudinal view, color Doppler delineates the true lumen during systole (lower left) and identifies a severe aortic regurgitation during diastole with a large jet at its origin (lower right, arrowhead). *Ao* true lumen of the ascending aorta

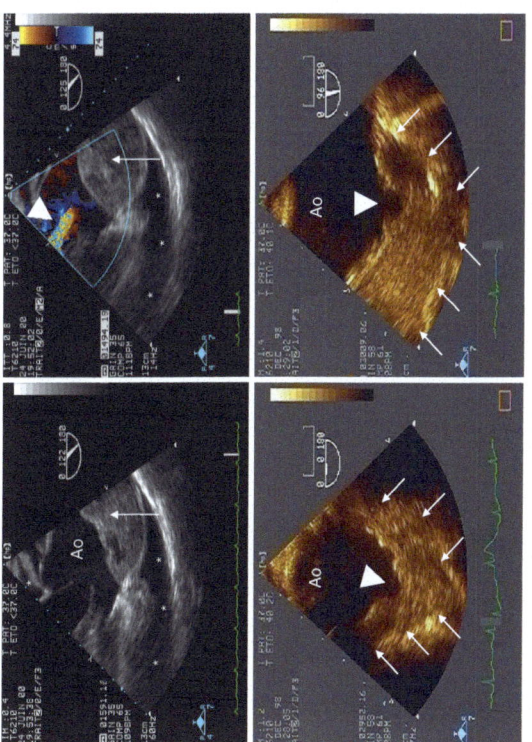

FIGURE 26.5 Transesophageal echocardiography performed in two patients ventilated for severe shock with suspected acute aortic syndrome. In the first patient, the mid-esophageal longitudinal view of the ascending aorta depicts a dilated vessel with a thickened wall consistent with a recent intramural hematoma (upper panels, arrow), a hemopericardium (asterisks), and color Doppler identifies a moderate aortic regurgitation (arrowhead). In the second patient, transesophageal echocardiography depicts a penetrating atherosclerotic ulcer of the descending thoracic aorta (lower panels, arrowhead) associated with a large hemomediastinum as an extravasation sign (arrows) Ao, aortic lumen

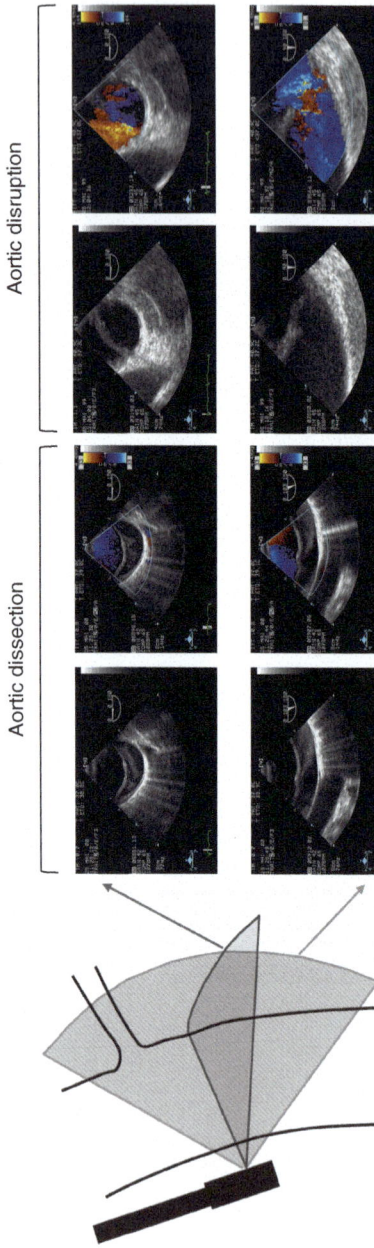

FIGURE 26.6 Differential transesophageal echocardiography findings which allow distinguishing the acute dissection from the traumatic disruption of the descending thoracic aorta in both the transverse (upper panels) and longitudinal (lower panels) views of the aortic isthmus. The intimal flap of the dissection is thin (mobile in real time) and extended, almost parallel to aortic walls in the longitudinal view, whereas the medial flap related to torn aortic wall is thick (nearly immobile in real time) and confined within a few centimeters, almost perpendicular to aortic walls in the longitudinal view. Color Doppler mapping depicts higher blood flow velocities in the true lumen of the dissected aorta (the noncirculating false lumen is here even partially thrombosed), while blood flow velocities are similar on both sides of the medial flap of the disrupted aorta (in this case, aliasing denotes turbulences in the surroundings of the traumatic aortic disruption)

TABLE 26.2 Differential transesophageal echocardiographic findings associated with aortic disruption and aortic dissection

Parameters to consider	Aortic dissection	Aortic disruption
Two dimensional echocardiography:		
• Aortic size:	• Increased	• Normal or increased
• Aortic contour:	• Symmetrical	• Asymmetrical (false aneurysm formation)
• Aortic flap:	• Thin (intimal), mobile • Extended (according to anatomical type), parallel to aortic walls	• Thick (medial), less mobile • Confined to the aortic isthmus, almost perpendicular to aortic walls
• Spatial extension: Number of aortic lumens:	• Two	• One
• Thrombus:	• Possible in false lumen	• None
• Extravasation signs:	• Possible (hemopericardium, rarely hemothorax)	• Possible (hemomediastinum, hemothorax)
Doppler:		
Color Doppler mapping:	• Distinct blood flow velocities (lower in the false channel)	• Similar blood flow velocities on both sides of the medial flap
	• Entry or reentry tear	• None
	• Obstruction of true lumen (compression by false lumen)	• Pseudo-coarctation (protrusion of disrupted aortic wall in lumen)
• Spectral Doppler.	• Identification of true lumen (pulse wave)	• Quantification of pressure gradient (continuous wave)

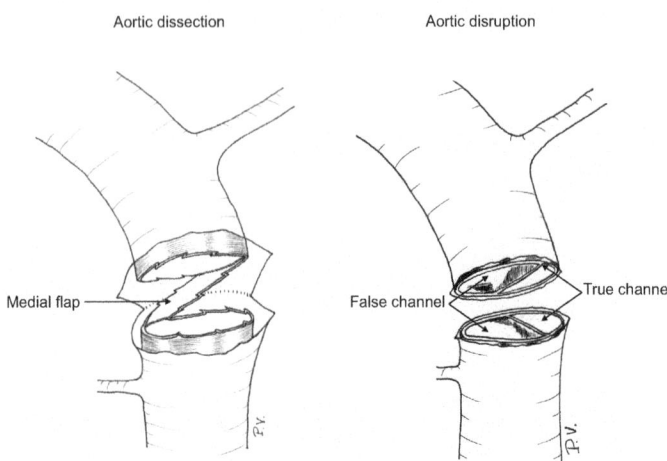

FIGURE 26.7 Schematic illustration of acute aortic dissection and traumatic aortic disruption with the adventitial layer artificially opened at the level of the aortic isthmus. Aortic dissection is characterized by a thin intimal flap that delimitates two distinct channels, whereas aortic disruption results in an intimal-medial flap that corresponds to a narrow band of aortic wall securing disrupted aortic segments a few centimeters apart. As a result, this medial flap fails to delimit two distinct channels

Multiple Choice Questions

1. In a patient with suspected acute dissection of the ascending aorta and circulatory failure, transthoracic echocardiography should be used to search for:

    A. A pericardial effusion
    B. A regional wall motion abnormality
    C. An enlarged ascending aorta
    D. An intimal flap within the aortic root
    E. An aortic insufficiency
    Answers: A, B, C, D, E

2. In patients with suspected acute aortic syndrome, transesophageal echocardiography should be used:

   A. Systematically as a first-line imaging technique
   B. In the subset of patients with hemodynamic instability who are mechanically ventilated
   C. To obtain additional information on the underlying causative aortic disease
   D. To diagnose cardiac tamponade in a spontaneously breathing patient
   E. Per-operatively to guide the emergency surgical procedure

   Answers: B, C, E

3. Transesophageal echocardiographic findings associated with subadventitial traumatic rupture of the aortic isthmus are:

   A. An extended intimal flap separating two distinct channels
   B. A medial flap confined within a few centimeters in the region of the aortic isthmus
   C. A false aneurysm formation of various size
   D. A posterior hemomediastinum
   E. The presence of similar blood flow velocities on both sides of the medial flap

   Answers: B, C, D, E

References

1. Vignon P, Guéret P, Vedrinne JM, Lagrange P, Cornu E, Abrieu O, Gastinne H, Bensaid J, Lang RM. Role of transesophageal echocardiography in the diagnosis and management of traumatic aortic disruption. Circulation. 1995;92(10):2959–68.
2. Vignon P, Martaillé JF, François B, Rambaud G, Gastinne H. Transesophageal echocardiography and therapeutic management of patients sustaining blunt aortic injuries. J Trauma. 2005;58(6):1150–8.

3. Vignon P, Boncoeur MP, François B, Rambaud G, Maubon A, Gastinne H. Comparison of multiplane transesophageal echocardiography and contrast-enhanced helical CT in the diagnosis of blunt traumatic cardiovascular injuries. Anesthesiology. 2001;94(4):615–22.

Suggested Readings

Erbel R, Aboyans V, Boileau C, Bossone E, Bartolomeo RD, Eggebrecht H, Evangelista A, Falk V, Frank H, Gaemperli O, Grabenwöger M, Haverich A, Iung B, Manolis AJ, Meijboom F, Nienaber CA, Roffi M, Rousseau H, Sechtem U, Sirnes PA, Allmen RS, Vrints CJ; ESC Committee for Practice Guidelines. 2014 ESC Guidelines on the diagnosis and treatment of aortic diseases: Document covering acute and chronic aortic diseases of the thoracic and abdominal aorta of the adult. The Task Force for the Diagnosis and Treatment of Aortic Diseases of the European Society of Cardiology (ESC). Eur Heart J. 2014;35(41):2873–926.
Vignon P, Spencer KT, Rambaud G, Preux PM, Krauss D, Balasia B, Lang RM. Differential transesophageal echocardiographic diagnosis between linear artifacts and intraluminal flap of aortic dissection or disruption. Chest. 2001;119(6):1778–90.

The manufacturer's authorised representative in the EU is Springer
Nature Customer Service Centre GmbH, Europaplatz 3, 69115 Heidelberg,
Germany. If you have any concerns regarding our products, please
contact ProductSafety@springernature.com

Printed and bound by CPI Group (UK) Ltd, Croydon, CR0 4YY
29/04/2026
02099519-0001